COMMUNICATION SKILLS
FOR VISUALLY IMPAIRED LEARNERS

COMMUNICATION SKILLS
FOR VISUALLY IMPAIRED LEARNERS

By

RANDALL K. HARLEY, Ph.D.

Professor, Special Education
George Peabody College for Teachers
of Vanderbilt University
Nashville, Tennessee

MILA B. TRUAN, Ed.D.

Reading Specialist
Tennessee School for the Blind
Nashville, Tennessee

LARHEA D. SANFORD, Ed.D.

Lead Teacher, Vision Program
Metropolitan Nashville Public School System
Nashville, Tennessee

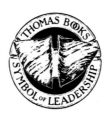

CHARLES C THOMAS • PUBLISHER
Springfield • Illinois • U.S.A.

Published and Distributed Throughout the World by

CHARLES C THOMAS • PUBLISHER

2600 South First Street

Springfield, Illinois 62794-9265

© *1987 by* CHARLES C THOMAS • PUBLISHER

ISBN 0-398-05364-2

Library of Congress Catalog Card Number: 87-10098

With THOMAS BOOKS *careful attention is given to all details of manufacturing and
design. It is the Publisher's desire to present books that are satisfactory as to their physical
qualities and artistic possibilities and appropriate for their particular use.* THOMAS
BOOKS *will be true to those laws of quality that assure a good name and good will.*

Printed in the United States of America

Q-R-3

Library of Congress Cataloging in Publication Data

Harley, Randall K.
    Communication skills for visually impaired learners.

    Bibliography: p.
    Includes index.
    1. Visually handicapped — Means of communication.
I. Truan, Mila B. II. Sanford, LaRhea. III. Title.
HV1631.5.H37   1987   371.91'1   87-10098
ISBN 0-398-05364-2

PREFACE

THIS BOOK is designed to provide a foundation for a better understanding of the teaching of communication skills to children, youth, and adults with visual impairment. The book is intended for use by teachers who have a basic knowledge of the skills for teaching communication skills to sighted pupils and who have a proficiency in reading and writing the braille literary code. A basic, fundamental understanding of the procedures for teaching communication skills should assist teachers and communication specialists who are concerned with helping the child with visual impairment to communicate at a level commensurate with the child's ability. Knowledge of the procedures for teaching braille communication skills will help the teacher of children who are visually impaired to have a healthy respect for a reading medium that has been used well over a 100 years.

This book has borrowed heavily from an earlier edition of *The Teaching of Braille Reading* by the authors with Freda M. Henderson. However, in this book the authors have endeavored to expand the scope of the communication skills to include the teaching of print reading to students who are visually impaired, as well as other communication skills, such as handwriting, braille writing, typing, listening and technology. After expanding the scope of the communications skills curriculum, the authors have added two chapters to help individualize communications skills for many students with visual impairment and special learning problems. In addition to enlarging the scope of this book, the authors have sought to update the teaching of communication skills with the latest technology which is available for teaching communication skills.

This book, *Communication Skills for Visually Impaired Learners,* is designed to update the research and to provide a more detailed explanation of the teaching methods which are unique to communication skills. Chapter 1 provides the historical perspectives of communication skills for students who are visually impaired, including braille and print reading, the written communication skills of handwriting, and listening. Chapter 2 describes the unique characteristics of reading readiness as related to the teaching of children who are visually impaired. Chapter 3 relates how three popular approaches to teaching reading can be used with these children. The main purpose of Chapter 4 is to alert teachers to the unique characteristics of teaching word identification skills to readers of braille and large print. In Chapter 5, the authors relate the uniqueness of assessment of reading skills of children who are visually impaired. They discuss the selection of tests and assessment techniques including formal and informal procedures. In Chapter 6, the purpose is to identify the characteristics of students who are visually impaired and who are having difficulty with learning problems meeting their potential. Chapter 7 identifies the methods and materials that vision specialists may try with students who are visually impaired with learning problems. Chapter 8 is designed to discuss aspects of writing that are unique to learners who are visually impaired, such as handwriting for low vision students, signature writing for blind students, braille writing, and typing skills.

Listening has become a very important communication skill for children who are visually impaired. Increased numbers of children who are visually impaired are now using listening as their primary means of gaining information from academic materials in school. In Chapter 9, readiness for listening, measurement of listening ability, teaching of listening skills, and improvement of listening speed are discussed. In Chapter 10, the use of braille reading with late blinded persons is discussed. These communication skills in braille reading may begin with practical skills such as reading watches, signs, playing cards, and labels. Unique approaches with older persons are discussed, such as the use of jumbo braille for persons with decreased tactual sensitivity. In Chapter 11, current technology in teaching of communication skills with learners who are visually impaired is discussed. Advances in technology have made many devices which help reduce the impact of visual handicaps in communication skills. Microcomputers and appropriate access equipment along with the use of closed-circuit TV, voice synthesizers, and electronic braille word processing are discussed. Chapter 12 deals with the selection of appropriate instructional materials and games which can help the teacher design individual education programs for children who are visually impaired. Guidelines are given for the selection of instructional materials.

The content of the book is based upon many years of experience by the authors in the actual teaching of students who are visually impaired in regular classes or in special remedial programs. It is hoped that the beginning teacher, as well as the experienced teacher, will find material and ideas in this book which can be helpful in the designing of communication skills instruction, and that all children and adults with visual impairment can have a successful and happy experience in the development of communication skills.

The authors wish to express their appreciation to several people who contributed to the preparation of this text. Special recognition is extended to Freda Henderson who was a major contributor to *The Teaching of Braille Reading* on which this textbook is based. The chapters titled "Reading in Perspective," "Approaches to Reading Instruction," and "Building Tactual Perception," were her major contributions to that work. The impact of her work as an author, researcher, college instructor, and elementary supervisor continues to serve professionals in the field and especially the authors of this book. We credit the Language Arts Committee at the Tennessee School for the Blind for the development of the instructional objectives in Appendixes B, C, & F. Billy Watson and Marietta Howington made valuable editorial suggestions. Appreciation is extended to students who used drafts of the manuscript and made helpful comments. We also wish to thank Muriel Sherwood for her contribution in typing and editing the many drafts of this edition. To the students with visual impairments who appear in the photographs illustrating the use of instructional materials, we express our sincere appreciation.

Randall K. Harley
Mila B. Truan
LaRhea D. Sanford

CONTENTS

COMMUNICATION SKILLS
FOR VISUALLY IMPAIRED LEARNERS

CHAPTER 1

HISTORICAL PERSPECTIVES

T HE FORMAL instruction of communication skills to visually impaired persons was initiated in 1784 when Valentine Hauy established the first school for the blind in Paris. Before Hauy, the learning of communication skills was largely a matter of learning to use listening skills or self-instruction using a tactual code devised by the blind person, himself. A brief history of the development of communication skills among blind persons can be divided into four areas: embossed reading, print reading, handwriting, and listening. Of these four areas, the literature on embossed reading is by far the most extensive.

EMBOSSED READING

Didymus of Alexandria is the first important recorded example of a blind person using a tactual reading form (French, 1932). Didymus won some reputation as a theologian and teacher during the fourth century. Although he obtained most of his material through listening and used many readers to read material to him, he was known to have used an alphabet carved in wood to learn to read.

In the early sixteenth century, Francisco Luces of Laragossa, Spain developed a set of letters carved on thin tablets of wood (Best, 1919). In 1651, George Harsdorffer of Nurenburg, Germany recommended cutting letters with a stylus on wax-coated tablets (Best, 1919). Blind Jacob of Netra, a village of Hesse in Germany, lived about the middle of the eighteenth century (French, 1932). He used a communication system of notches cut with his knife in small sticks. Jacob accumulated a small library of books consisting of bundles of notched sticks.

In "An Essay on Blindness" written prior to 1773, M. Diderot related a visit to a blind man. He said, "It was about five in the afternoon when we came to the blind man's house, where we found him hearing his blind son read with raised characters" (Illingworth, 1910, p. 4). Maria Theresia von Pardis, born in 1759, was known for marking her playing cards with pinpricks, tangible in relief (French, 1932). She also represented letters by sticking pins in a large pincushion. Other blind persons devised their own kinds of tactual systems to record material that they may have felt would be hard to memorize. Among these earlier systems of communication were the following: (1) knots on a string, (2) cut paper letters on threads in the form of words, (3) carved wooden letters, (4) movable letters cast in lead or tin, (5) letters marked with a blunt instrument on wax-coated tablets, (6) letters cut out of cardboard, (7) pinpricked letters on paper, and (8) embossed print letters on paper.

Valentine Hauy secured information on reading and writing from Maria von Paradis on a visit to Paris about 1784 (French, 1932). He began teaching his first pupil, Francois Lesueur, to read letters of the alphabet which were carved on thin wooden tablets (Lowenfeld, 1975). In 1786, Lesueur first detected the outlines of a letter that had been strongly impressed in a print funeral notice. In fact, it was the "0" in the funeral notice that caught his attention (Best, 1919). In his early experiments with teaching blind persons, Hauy noticed that he could teach Lesueur to read letters that had been embossed on wet paper through a printing press. He soon taught this young blind man to read embossed letters, and embossed letters became the mode of the day for blind students learning to read.

Hauy employed a line italic type letter that was very large (Illingworth, 1910). In fact, it took 365 characters for 50 square inches. In comparison with Hauy's letter, James Gall of Edinburgh could emboss 526 characters in a space of the same size. Samual Gridley Howe's first Boston line letter was small enough so that 702, and later, 1,067 characters could fit into a 50 inch square (Best, 1919). The Boston line letter was adopted by the American Association of Instructors for the Blind in 1853 (AAIB, 1853).

The Raised Line systems soon had competition from raised dot systems of communication. In 1808, a Frenchman, Charles Barbier, contributed a paper entitled "Ecriture Nocturne" to the French Academy of Sciences (French, 1932). Barbier, an officer in Napoleon's army, was attempting to develop a method of sending coded military messages that could be read "under cover of darkness." Barbier developed a 2 x 6 dot cell which could be embossed in a metal writing frame which is a forerunner of the modern slate and stylus. Barbier's system was exhibited in 1820 at the School for the Blind in Paris. Louis Braille, a pupil at the school, liked the dot system much better than the raised line letters, but Louis felt that the elongated cell was too long to fit under the fingertips, and he devised a 6-dot 3 × 2 cell which was more suitable for the finger. He devised a braille music notations system before designing a braille alphabet. In 1829, Louis Braille published his dot code which is very much like the highly organized and systematic arrangement of the braille code that is in use today (French, 1932). The upper cell configuration used in the first 10 letters of the alphabet is repeated in systematic fashion for the other letters of the braille alphabe, as noted in Figure 1.

ENGLISH BRAILLE CHARACTERS

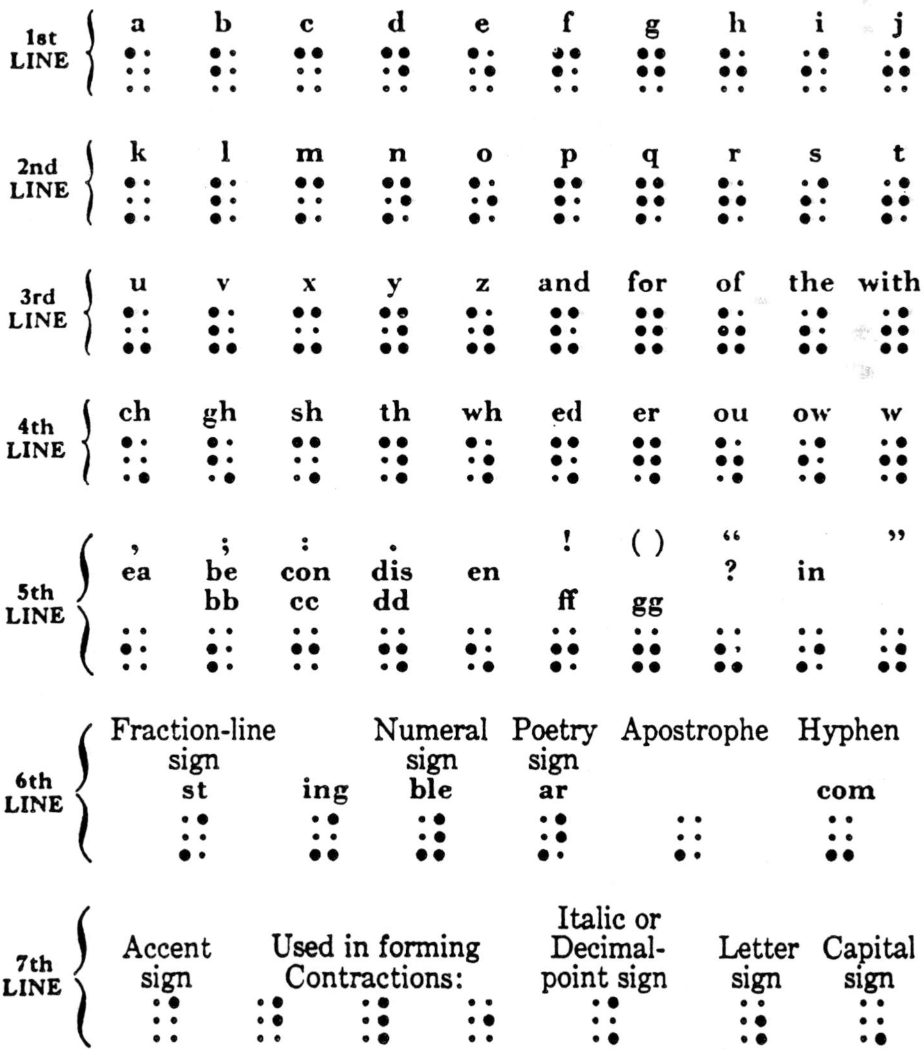

1st LINE	a	b	c	d	e	f	g	h	i	j
2nd LINE	k	l	m	n	o	p	q	r	s	t
3rd LINE	u	v	x	y	z	and	for	of	the	with
4th LINE	ch	gh	sh	th	wh	ed	er	ou	ow	w
5th LINE	, ea	; be bb	: con cc	. dis dd	en	! ff	( ) gg	" ?	in	"
6th LINE	Fraction-line sign st	ing	Numeral sign ble	Poetry sign ar	Apostrophe	Hyphen com
7th LINE	Accent sign	Used in forming Contractions:			Italic or Decimal-point sign	Letter sign	Capital sign

Figure 1. Standard English Braille, Grade 2

The first slate or writing frame for embossing dots was designed by Charles Barbier with a 12-dot cell. Louis Braille used the Barbier slate for his 6-dot cell by covering up six of the lower dots. Barbier's writing frame consisted of two parts between which the paper was placed (French, 1932). Depressions for the dots were indented in a wooden board. A wood or metal guide was placed over the wooden board and paper was perforated with a blunt-pointed steel instrument.

In the meantime, the raised line letter introduced by Valentine Hauy had been introduced in schools for the blind in other European countries. In 1822, Edmond Fry of London offered a prize for the best line letter system. In 1827, James Gall of Edinburgh (Best, 1919) issued his first book for teaching the art of reading to the blind. In this book he used a raised print character for a regular Roman alphabet, using triangular or angular letters of lower case forms. In 1832, Samuel Gridley Howe used raised line letters at Perkins Institute for the Blind in Watertown, Massachusetts. He later became known as the developer of the Boston Line Type which was used in several American schools for the blind. Dr. Howe's letters consisted entirely of lower case letters of angular type. In 1833, The Gospel of Mark was embossed in raised print at the Pennsylvania Institute for the Instruction of the Blind in Philadelphia (Best, 1919). This gospel was the first book for the blind embossed in America. In 1835, Howe printed the Book of Acts and in 1936 the entire New Testament.

In 1837, J. H. Frere of Black Heath, London used a phonetic system of stenographic and angular forms which were sharply defined for touch (Best, 1919). This raised line letter system became popular in Great Britain. In 1847, Dr. William Moon of Brighton, England devised a modified form of Frere's system based on regular type (Best, 1919) Some of his forms were outlines of letters and some consisted of angles, half circles, and straight lines. Both Frere and Moon used return line reading, that is, one line was read left to right and the next line right to left. Frere revised his characters in the return line but Moon did not use reversals (Illingworth, 1910).

The Moon system which became very popular for late-blinded adults is still used today, largely in Great Britain. This form is the only popularly used raised line system, and a number of books have been reproduced in this form. The Fishburne alphabet (Newman & Hall, 1986), using a system of both lines and dots, was developed for use by late-blinded adults in labeling foods and medicines. The other embossed forms of communication for the blind have largely used various kinds of dot systems.

In 1860, a form of braille was adopted for the first time in the United States at the Missouri School for the Blind (French, 1932). In 1868, William Wait of New York Institute for the Blind introduced New York Point, a system probably developed by Dr. John D. Russ (Illingworth, 1910). This dot system, using a cell 2 dots high with a variable base of 1, 2, 3, and 4 dots in width, sometimes was used across 2 cells. This overlapping of cells was made possible by the narrow metal vertical strip between each cell of the slate or metal guide. New York Point was endorsed and recommended for use in American schools by the American Association of Instructors for the Blind in 1871 (Irwin, 1955).

An early method of writing New York Point braille and embossed script was to impress it by means of a stylus on paper placed over a soft background such as baize, rubber, or soft leather (Illingworth, 1910). The guide for the stylus was made of a strip of brass containing one or two lines of oblong holes of the required size.

Joel W. Smith in 1878 introduced a modified braille code at Perkins Institute for the Blind (Illingworth, 1910). This modified American Braille was the forerunner of the braille system used in the United States in later years, and was modeled after the braille system used in Great Britain. During the latter part of the 19th Century and the early part of the 20th Century, a battle developed in America over the use of New York Point and the American Braille system. Most Midwestern and South Atlantic schools used the New York Point system embossed at the American Printing House for the Blind, and most New England schools used the American Braille embossed at Howe Press. In the 1910 census, blind persons in the United States were using five types of embossed print: New York Point, American Braille, English Braille, Line Point, and Moon Type. The account of the "battle" of the dot system in America can be obtained from *As I Saw It* by Robert Irwin (1955).

In 1913 (Best, 1919), the American Association of Workers for the Blind Uniform Type Committee recommended Standard Dot Braille over either American Braille or New York Point. Standard Dot was a system using the 3 × 2 cell but having less contractions than the British system. Standard Dot later became known as Grade 1 1/2 braille. In 1932, the Americans and British agreed upon a Grade 2 braille by the American Printing House for the Blind, the Library of Congress, the American Association of Workers for the Blind, and the American Association of Instructors for the Blind. This committee, called the Joint Uniform Braille Committee, was made up of members appointed by the professional associations for workers and teachers of the blind.

Among the important historical influences on the embossed system used in the United States have been the developments of federal subsidies for the embossing of books. In 1858, the American Printing House was established at Louisville, Kentucky (Best, 1919). At first, this was a cooperative group of residential schools using the basement of the Ketucky School for the Blind to emboss books for blind pupils. Later, in March of 1879 the American Printing House was subsidized by an Act of Congress through the first federal legislation providing money for education of handicapped children. This subsidy granted $10,000 annually for the publication of embossed books and the manufacture of tangible apparatus. The American Printing House for the Blind continues to be subsidized but in a much larger amount by the Congress of the United States, and children who are registered at the American Printing House for the Blind can obtain materials on quota, such as braille books, large print books, or braille writers and other tangible apparatus. In 1913, Congress enacted legislation requiring that the American Printing House for the Blind deposit in the Library of Congress a copy of every embossed book (Farrell, 1956). Since then the Library of Congress services have been expanded to include records, cassette tapes, large print materials, etc.

One of the major developments that helped popularize the use of braille instead of New York Point was the development in 1892 of a mechanical braille writer. This embosser which operated much like a typewriter was developed by Frank Hall, Superintendent of the Illinois Braille and Sight-Saving School (French, 1932). This invention and his braille stereotype machine (for making metal plates for embossing pages of books) did much to make braille more popular, even though a counterpart was made for New York Point braille by William Wait, Superintendent of the New York Institute for the Blind. Wait's machine, the Kleidograph, though operable by one hand was not a simple machine and was not nearly as strong and durable as the Hall braille writer. The inventions by Hall helped to establish the 2×3 dot cell as the dominant pattern of embossed writing.

Braille writers are now manufactured in the United States, Germany, The Netherlands, France, Japan, Great Britain, and India. The computer controlled embossers are manufactured in the United States, Norway, The Netherlands, France, and Germany. Stereotypes and duplicators for braille are manufactured in the United States, Great Britain, Germany, Japan, Sweden, and India (Gill, 1983).

Problems with the use of braille books have been primarily the excessive storage space and the speed of reading. In order to overcome the storage problem, a paperless braille writer has been developed to help reduce storage space. It is also helpful in word processing for blind persons desiring to emboss materials in braille. Special instructional programs have helped to improve reading speed, but slow reading speeds continue to be a problem in the education of the visually impaired. The increased use of listening materials has helped improve speed in obtaining information. Other problems have been the producing of satisfactory mathematical and music codes. The teaching of braille to adults and developmentally delayed children has always been a problem in the use of braille materials. The use of braille with children below an intelligence quotient of 85 has been discouraged (Nolan & Kederis, 1969).

The integration of blind children in day school programs has greatly increased the demand for many kinds of instructional books and materials in braille. In recent years, technology has helped to produce braille books by the use of computers. Some efforts have been attempted (Foulke, 1979) to change the code by increasing the number of dots, especially for the many symbols needed in braille mathematical and scientific materials. Even the abandoning of braille itself has been a threat to some blind persons, and the BRAILLE REVIVAL LEAGUE has been established to ensure that braille receives proper emphasis in schools and rehabilitation programs.

The number of braille users among the legally blind registrants at the American Printing House for the Blind continues to remain a small percentage of the total number of registrants. In the 1985 registration (American Printing House, 1986), braille readers formed only 15% of the total group. However, visual readers of 36%, auditory readers at 23%, and pre-readers and non-readers at 26% were all larger groups of these registrants.

PRINT READING

In 1908, Dr. N. Bishop Harman established the world's first school for partially seeing in London. In 1909, Robert Irwin opened a class for blind children in Cleveland, Ohio and in 1910 he enrolled two children with "defective vision" (Frampton & Rowell, 1938). In 1910, C.A. Hamilton, Superintendent of the New York School for the Blind in Batavia reported that some of the partially seeing pupils from his school had joined regular classes in Batavia High School (Hamilton, 1910). In September of 1911, Fanny S. Fletcher started the first sight-saving classes in Detroit (Frampton

& Kerney, 1953). In 1909, Edward E. Allen, Director of Perkins Institute and Massachusetts School for the Blind, learned of the newly established London school for partially seeing children while attending a near-by conference, and in 1913 a class for partially seeing children was opened in Roxbury, Massachusetts. Soon classes for partially seeing children were established in the public school systems of Cleveland, Chicago, Milwaukee, and New York. Although most of these early classes were segregated classes, a cooperative plan was developed in Cleveland whereby the partially seeing children undertook work requiring special teaching equipment in their special classroom, but they participated with the normally seeing pupils in some activities, such as oral work.

The first classes of partially seeing children were based on the philosophy of sight conservation. Teachers were trained to use techniques which would save the sight of their children. Their classes were called "sight-saving" classes, "conservation of vision" classes or classes for the "semi-sighted" (Van Cleave, 1916). A popular notion was that vision could be saved like money in a bank. Even schools for the visually impaired were named braille and "sight-saving" schools. Their children were encouraged to gain information through their senses other than the visual sense. Even children with large amounts of residual vision were taught to read braille in order to conserve their sight. The assumption was that the use of the child's limited vision would destroy what vision remained. The barriers to the use of vision of partially seeing and low vision children have largely come from the myth that using the eyes causes further damage, whereas, limited use would save the vision and protect the child from further impairment. Sight utilization rather than sight-saving has been emphasized by the teachers of the visually impaired since the 1960s and 1970s.

Most visually impaired children have enough remaining vision to read ink print of some form. In recent years, medical specialists have increasingly emphasized the importance of using vision rather than saving it. The research by Barraga (1964) and others showed that vision was not lost, but visual efficiency was improved through use and training. Research has been followed by changes in educational practice. Reports of registration of legally blind children at the American Printing House for the Blind from 1961 to 1985 has shown a decline in the percentage of children reading braille and an increase in the percentage of children reading print.

The size of print in large print books has been decreasing since the early 1900s. Large print books were first introduced by Irwin in the

Cleveland Public School in 1913 (Eakin & McFarland, 1960). These books were printed in 36-point clear faced type (72 points equal 1 inch), as illustrated in Figure 2. Soon 24-point type proved most legible among partially seeing children in the Cleveland Schools. Nolan (1959) found no significant differences in reading speed between 18-point and 24-point type sizes. Large print textbooks are now mostly produced in 18-point type at the American Printing House for the Blind. Birch, Tisdall, Peabody, & Sterrett (1966), studying the relationships of type size to achievement of partially seeing children, found that no one type size can be considered superior to others. Individual differences among the children indicated that some children do best in each of several sizes, ranging from 12 to 24 points.

Type is measured in points from the bottom of the lowest letter (for example, the tail of the letter *y*) to the top of the tallest capital; type an inch high measures 72 points. Most adult books are set in 10- to 12-point type, newspapers are often 8 point, and some editions of the Bible are in 6-point type. By comparison, 14-point type is considered the minimum size for large-type materials. Large-type materials are most commonly available in 16- to 18-point type size.

Samples of Type

This is 12 point type.

This is 14 point type.

This is 18 point type.

This is 24 point type.

This is 30 point type.

This is 36 point type.

Figure 2. Common Type Sizes

Less attention has been given to the style of print, the thickness of the letters and spacing between the letters and line of print. However, a heavy serif-type print called "clearface" was used in the 36-point type books in 1914.

In 1920, a research study with children showed that a 24-point type called "Caslon Bold" was superior to six different type faces presented in various point sizes (Eakin & MacFarland, 1960). "Clear type" books were published for partially seeing children until 1942. Since 1946, pages of existing books have been photographed to give enlargement without resetting the type.

A more recent trend is to use regular size print with optical aids. Many children can read just as rapidly using optical aids with regular print as with large print alone. Reading speeds with textbooks in large print have been compared with reading speeds for standard print when suitable optical aids were used. Sykes (1971) and Sloan and Habel (1973) found that visually impaired students performed as well in using 12-point type and using optical aids as they did with 18-point print without optical aids.

HANDWRITING

A variety of methods to teach handwriting to blind students can be found in the early history of education of the blind. Valentine Hauy and his contemporaries used a stylus to make characters in a reversed form on a sheet of paper placed upon felt, rubber, or some other substance (Illingworth, 1910). Writing was done right to left, similar to the way the writing on a braille slate is done today. Hauy also used glutenous ink to write boldly upon paper. Over this he sprinkled sand which adhered to the letters to form a rough form of relief writing. He also encouraged his pupils to write with a very stiff steel pen on paper placed over a soft material so that the indentations could be read on the reverse side. James Gall used a little strip of brass with square openings in which the Roman characters were formed by the writer (Illingworth, 1910). Dr. William Moon used paper crossed with raised lines to teach handwriting. Typewriting paper was placed over the grooved cardboard with paper clips. Later, screen wire was used with paper and a crayon to raise the letters off the paper enough to be detected by the finger. Another procedure was to use thin twine stretched tightly across the face of an ordinary braille slate clipboard in lines about half an inch apart and later glued to the board. The twine was felt through the paper by the blind writer (Illingworth, 1910).

In a residential school for the blind, writing with a lead pencil was taught by placing the paper upon corrugated cardboard containing a number of parallel grooves in which the bodies of the letters were formed in order that they might be of uniform sizes. The grooves could be felt through the paper. The grooves also served to keep the lines straight and equidistant. "By this method of writing most of our pupils correspond with their parents and friends" (Tennessee School for theBlind, 1877, p. 306).

Another system of writing consisted of point-writing or pricking through firm glazed paper with a stylus. The relative position of the dots made on the other side of the paper was used to make the different letters of the alphabet (Tennesse School for the Blind, 1877).

Two forms of handwriting have been prevalent in the early history of schools for the blind in the United States. Square handwriting was initiated at Perkins by 1837. Laura Bridgman's daily journal was started in square handwriting in 1841 and was continued throughout her life (Farrell, 1956). Round handwriting was used at Perkins before 1837, and later at the New York Institute in 1936. Modern technology has helped handwriting through the provision of such devices as closed circuit television and special writing boards and kits.

LISTENING

Listening has been an important tool of communication for blind persons long before embossed communication was developed. The blind soothsayers of ancient China and India showed that some blind persons could become "walking libraries" without being literate in the traditional sense of being able to read and write. Didymus of Alexandria gained his knowledge through listening to special readers (French, 1932). "So great was his zeal and endurance that he frequently tired his readers out," "He meditated much on what he heard, read and thus gained a clear idea of the meaning of passages" (p. 66). His scholarship led to an appointment as professor at the Institute of Higher Learning in Alexandria. Nicholas Saunderson used listening to become a professor of math at Cambridge long before embossed writing was developed for the blind.

Listening was a very important means of obtaining information in the early residential schools. Teachers of the blind were often caught between the confusion of embossed types (New York Point, Boston Line Print, and Braille). In regard to the 1870s, Hendrickson (1972) states for the Illinois Braille and Sight-Saving School, "In the last years of Rhoade's administration there has been a trend back to reliance on oral instruction, largely because there were few purchases of reading materials."

The limited availability of embossed materials also encouraged oral instruction at the Tennessee School for the Blind in the 1870s. "Instruction was given in the remaining studies orally, and with aid of such books in raised print as could be obtained. The whole number of books as get published in raised letters will scarcely exceed eight or ten times the amount of reading matter contained in the Bible. Of these some are out of print, and some are of little value on account of their clumsy and complicated typography" (Tennessee School for the Blind, 1877, p. 306).

The reading of raised letters was much slower than the reading of raised dots. The reading of raised dots was slow enough. Hayes (1918, 1920) found a mean reading rate of about 64 words per minute among blind readers. Even in 1969, braille reading rates were 72 words per minute (residential school) as compared to 84 words per minute (day school) at the fourth grade level (Lowenfeld, Abel, & Hatlen, 1969). The slowness of braille reading and the difficulty of braille for multihandicapped or adventitiously blinded adults has also helped to place a heavy emphasis on listening as the mode for obtaining information for blind persons.

Dictaphone records were used in the early classes for blind children in Cleveland and Minneapolis. The American Foundation for the Blind estimated in 1932 that not more than 10% of the blind population were sufficient in tactual reading to enjoy embossed books. The Foundation helped to develop a phonograph disc that played at 33 1/3 revolutions. This disc and its player was named a "Talking Book" and made available in 1934 (Farrell, 1956).

Since 1934, books on cassette or tape recorded materials have become much more popular than disc recorded books. In addition, the new technology of the late 20th Century has provided talking watches, calculators, measuring devices, elevators, cars, etc. that increased the importance of listening for blind persons. More important to the teacher are children's learning aids and microcomputers that talk to the listener. Reading machines that convert print into listening such as the Kurzweil (See chapter on technology) give hope to the visually impaired reader who looks to the future for more independence and less reliance on sighted readers.

SUMMARY

A brief review of the history of communication skills for the visually impaired shows that the description of the development of embossed reading for blind persons is by far the most extensive. After much trial and debate, the 6-dot cell is used in most parts of the world today.

The major development in the history of education of low vision persons has been a change in philosophy from sight-saving to sight utilization. Large print for low vision children has generally become smaller and more variable in size, especially with the large influx of optical aids. Listening was important at first because of lack of adequate materials in either embossed or print forms, and it continues to be important today because of lack of materials and because of the increased speed obtained from listening to recorded materials. The changes in the importance of listening skills have become more important through the advent of modern technology and the increase in school enrollments of multiply handicapped children. Handwriting techniques have progressed from relatively crude but innovative devices used in the early schools for the blind to more modern forms through the use of technology such as closed circuit television and the development of special raised line writing boards and kits.

CHAPTER 2

READING READINESS

READING READINESS training for visually impaired children is very similar in most respects to readiness training for sighted children. The training for most sighted children consists of activities of perception, auditory discrimination, and language development. Training for visually impaired students is expanded to include tactual perception as well. A number of research studies (Spache & Spache, 1973) can be cited which show that reading readiness training results in improved success in reading for young sighted children. Many young children may progress satisfactorily in reading without the formal readiness training. Superior ability or informal readiness training obtained at home helps to provide the necessary background of experience for the development of concepts, language, and interest in books.

Visually impaired children are at a special disadvantage in obtaining informal reading readiness training at home. Monroe (1951) listed the following concepts which children establish in their gradual development of awareness of books to actual reading:

1. Books contain pages to be turned.
2. Pictures resemble familiar objects.
3. Pictures and books have a top and bottom, front and back.
4. Books give information and pleasure.
5. Language is constant on each page.
6. Language can be remembered and related to specific pages or pictures.
7. Content of the book stimulates the child's own related ideas.
8. Printed symbols tell the reader what to say.

A special emphasis on pictures occurs in this developmental process. Visually impaired children are at a serious disadvantage with little or no input about the pictures. Other deficiencies caused by lack of vision are not so obvious. In this chapter the unique characteristics of reading readiness as related to teaching visually impaired children are emphasized.

CONCEPTUAL DEVELOPMENT

Probably the most apparent difference between readiness preparation of sighted children and visually impaired children is the emphasis on the development of all sensory processes. Most of the information about the environment for sighted children comes through the eyes and somewhat less through the ears. Vision is the unifying sense that gives overall meaning to the different information provided by each of the senses separately. Visually impaired children must learn to integrate the sensory impressions from all the senses through use of touch, hearing, smell, taste, and any remaining vision. These impressions are most accurate when they are the result of concrete experiences.

Cutsforth (1951) felt that blind children were taught to accept verbal descriptions of the sighted, but that they could attach little meaning to these descriptions because of a lack of concrete experience. Thus, blind children formed many misconceptions due to this lack of experience. For instance, a blind teacher who was teaching small blind children to read revealed to her pupils that cows were bigger than elephants for the teacher had never touched an elephant or a cow. Also, a third grade boy in a resource room for visually impaired children was having trouble finding any motivation to read a poem about a bird. His teacher discovered that he had never had the opportunity to touch a bird.

In a pilot study with eighteen visually impaired children between the ages of six and thirteen, Harley (1963) found that the greatest deficiencies in the concept areas occurred in words related to farm and nature and the least amount in items related to home and clothing. For example, these subjects had difficulty in identifying models and actual objects such as a duck, turkey, fish, squirrel, and rabbit; or plow, hoe, and tractor. The results of a larger study with forty blind children in the same age group showed that the children who are young, less intelligent or less experienced need to have far greater contact with their environment to form accurate concepts than children who are older, more intelligent and/or more experienced.

Visually impaired children are usually confined to a more restricted portion of their environment than seeing children. They are not as motivated to explore new objects beyond their reach or limited visual field. Without visual stimulation, they may lack the motivation to move out and examine their environment. Protective parents and teachers may further limit experiences by keeping the children at home or in a special classroom to prevent physical injury or failure. Fraiberg (1977) noted the prolonged period of immobility during the first year of life of young blind children. She noted that it was not until late in the first year of development that the totally blind children reached for an object on sound cue alone. In describing this delay in self-initiated mobility, she noted that sighted babies, who were reaching for objects by visual cue alone at six months, were not able to make the connection between the objects and the sound alone until near 12 months. The immobility for the blind babies posed a serious problem by limiting the exploration and discovery of objects in the environment.

The frequency of contact needed to become familiar with objects and to make generalizations about their environement can be a problem with visually impaired children. Normally seeing children have an advantage in this respect. For example, a normally seeing child will see fire engines racing down the street, inside the fire station, pictured in a book or on television, and have many opportunities to build a concept of the appearance and use of fire engines. The visually impaired children and the seeing children may make the same field trip to the fire station, but the visually impaired child will not have as complete an impression as the sighted child. First, because it is the blind child's only concrete or physical contact with a fire engine and, second, because there are important details about the fire engine that are only available through vision such as the unique color. The visually impaired children may not see the fire engine again until another trip is made to the station. They may be able to parrot words about the fire engine yet have a hazy concept about the characteristics of a fire engine. Even tactual exploration of the fire engine provides segmented information that may be loosely integrated. Verbal learning even with appropriate concrete experiences is thus a serious problem for young visually impaired children who are beginning to read (See Figure 3).

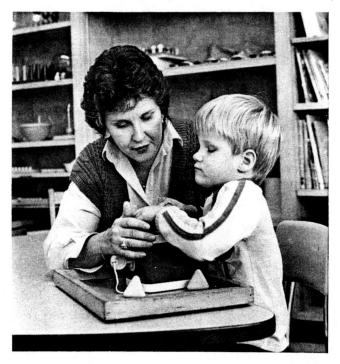

Figure 3. Verbal learning with appropriate concrete experience.

The range of experiences for totally blind children is restricted to a smaller portion of their environment than the range for normally seeing or even partially sighted children. Visually impaired children are restricted to the use of their remaining senses, i.e., feeling, listening, tasting, and smelling. Lacking vision, they must gain a concrete knowledge of their object world mostly by touch experiences. Lowenfeld (1973) showed how the tactual space perception of blind children is different from the visual space perception of seeing children. The basis for the difference is that tactual perception required direct contact with the object to be observed. This restriction greatly reduces the range and variety of experiences available because some items are too far away, too large, too small, too fragile, or too dangerous to handle. The sun, moon, and stars are too far away. The mountain or lake is too large to comprehend as a whole. The amoeba is so small that it must be viewed under a microscope. A spider web is too delicate to examine tactually without destroying it. Wild animals, fire, or a mixer blade are too dangerous to touch. Liquids in thermometers or needles on electronic instruments are inaccessible behind glass covers.

The teacher may help develop more accurate concepts, using concreteness in teaching by bringing a variety of items to school for the child to explore, and by encouraging children to engage in show-and-tell activities with items from their home. Real objects of full-scale representations are better than models. Models, however, may sometimes be very helpful in building concepts. The ideal reading readiness classroom is one that is full of materials, learning centers, projects, animals, plants, etc. which are used to provide the basis of concreteness for the curriculum. Field trips which are well-planned and integrated into units or teaching modules are essential in providing the needed concreteness. With this enrichment, reading becomes meaningful, exciting, and challenging to the young visually impaired child.

A teacher may be surprised that Johnny has not seen a rabbit when Johnny begins to read a story about a rabbit. The teacher will soon learn that Johnny can understand and enjoy the story about the rabbit much better after a rabbit is brought to school for Johnny to examine. The resourceful teacher of visually impaired children should provide many and varying concrete experiences for the children before beginning reading. Success in meaningful reading will depend largely on the background of experience of the readers. The visually impaired children's prior stock of impressions will determine in a large measure on how much meaning they will derive from the tactual or print symbols. Even if parents have exposed children to a variety of experiences, the teacher may discover many conceptual gaps.

Anne Sullivan Macy took Helen Keller out into the real world to learn. She learned the word "water" while pumping water over her hands, and she learned botany while sitting in a tree. A good readiness program will be exciting and interesting for the child using real life situations in a classroom that is not bounded by walls but takes advantage of the stimulation inherent in the natural world. A program that teaches reading to young blind children can be a program of freedom, excitement, and enjoyment. It can be a program of field trips, manipulative tasks, activities with plants and animals, of creative experiences, and of play. The child can learn about "potatoes" by planting, cultivating, harvesting, peeling, cutting, cooking, and eating them. The innovative teacher can look at pictures in the beginning reading readiness and pre-primer books, bring in materials, and dramatize activities that will make the stories more meaningful and more exciting to read. For example, a teacher in a primary grade reading group of children in a rural community found that they did not understand the concept of hanging clothes out to dry on a pulley arrangement for an upper floor apartment. This arrangement was pictured in the book and was essential to the plot of the story. She made the story more meaningful and exciting by bringing in two large appliance boxes, cutting windows in them, attaching pulleys and rope, and hanging clothes on them so that the children could pretend the activity themselves. This readiness activity took extra time and energy for the teacher but the pay-off was a stimulating, fun-type experience for the children that helped them to want to read the story.

Anderson and Olson (1981) found that young congenitally blind children (ages 3-10) assigned more egocentric (personal experiences) and many functional attributes to tangible objects (top, ball, pencil, key, etc.) than matched sighted children who used more perceptual attributes (color, shape, physical characteristics, etc.). In a comparison of congenitally blind and sighted children ages 3-9, Anderson (1984), concluded that the cognitive delays of the blind children resulted from the limited manner by which they experience the object world. In both studies it was concluded that blind children need more experience with real objects and more opportunity to understand the relationship between word-names and objects.

Hall and Rodabaugh (1979) developed a program of carefully sequenced, concrete experiences using a multisensory approach to learning in order to develop the concepts needed for reading. Of 200 relevant concepts identified, 32 were selected and lessons were designed to teach these concepts. The authors noted that very little knowledge was available concerning the developmental stages of concept acquisition in visually impaired children. The strengths of the program according to teachers in the field test were its ease of use, high interest level, and choice of concepts. However, teachers felt that a major weakness was the requirement that they collect a large number of concrete objects for use with the lessons; they preferred that the materials be provided in a pre-assembled kit.

The following list represents a continuum on a concreteness-abstractness scale for developing concepts related to extending the frame of reference for blind children, the most concrete listed first. It also represents a scale of desirability of tactual experience for visually impaired children. The more real and accurate the experience the better. It may be noted also that the more real an experience is, the less interpretation will be required of the teacher. The more abstract the experience, the more assistance the teacher will need to provide.

Tangible Aids Guide

- the child's own body (including self concepts and body concepts)
- the real object
- full scale, accurate representation of the object
- an accurate scale model, proportionate
- an accurate representation, three-dimensional
- stylized representation, three-dimensional
- two-dimensional representation
- symbolic representation
- analogical representation
- verbal description and discussion with the student, oral-aural (inactive)
- verbal description, oral (one-way)

LANGUAGE DEVELOPMENT

The development of meaningful receptive and expressive language in visually impaired children may require more time than with seeing children because of several factors:

1. Due to a lack of experience, the visually impaired child usually lacks many of the concepts needed to develop meaningful language. Because of blindness, mobility is more limited. Since the child is limited in moving about in the environment, experiences are limited.

2. The visually impaired child may lack or have little visual sensory input which limits experiences to perception primarily through the tactual and auditory senses. With limited or total loss of visual information, the child's tactual and auditory senses provide less information on which to build concepts for language development.

Delayed language development can affect reading success. Children with limited vocabularies, incomplete articulation, and limited ability to communicate cannot be expected to profit fully from reading instruction. The child with a very limited vocabulary cannot be expected to understand unfamiliar words written in braille or large print. Success in braille or print reading requires a basic understanding of words. Children whose language has incomplete articulation, abbreviated and incomplete sentences, omitted or distorted syllables, or scrambled word order are at a real disadvantage when learning to read and write. With such language differences, children cannot match the sounds and sequences of the words they speak with those written in books. Since a major strategy for successful reading and writing is predicting written language from spoken language, students with language differences are at a distinct disadvantage (Smith, 1978). The educational impact of racial and ethnic language differences has been substantially documented (Baratz & Shuy, 1969). Yet, the relationship between aberrant oral language and delays in learning to read and write by children who are visually impaired and racially or culturally different from their classmates has not been explored.

Conversation is the visually impaired child's earliest experience with language. In a conversation, words in phrases transmit the core of ideas. In conversation crucial information is provided by changes in pitch, rate, articulation, and volume. Often a child's preferred communication method is by tone of voice or intensity of feeling. The unhappy 2-year-old left by its mother with the sitter shows anger at being "abandoned" with a loud wail. The child is using tone and intensity of voice to communicate without words. Even though the child may have been able to articulate "Mama go" meaning that it wanted to go, too, the wail was the most basic and powerful attempt at communicating. Another component in communication for the sighted listener is provided by gestures and facial expressions. Considerable meaning may be learned from facial expressions and body language, even when words are unintelligible as when watching a movie in a foreign language.

Listening to television or records is the counterpart to reading because the listener and speaker have little or no interaction. In a conversation the listener and speaker swap roles repeatedly. Each can ask questions to test the correctness of impressions, which is not the case with listening to television. Then the listener, like the reader, must make an independent interpretation of what is read or heard. Spoken language and written language have elements in common as conveyers of thought through words, but words are sounds in spoken language and combination of letters in written language.

The processes by which children learn to listen and speak are uniquely different from the ways they learn to read and write. Children learn to understand what they hear primarily at home and from the family and other familiar persons. Children's first language concerns their primary needs from primary care givers, so that they have a natural motivation to communicate. First conversations are about immediate and significant occurrences. Language learning happens the entire time the child is awake and wherever the child is. Language in the home is not formally taught, but the child imitates what is heard. Parents at times correct the child's incorrect choice of words, articulation, ending of words, and completeness of meaning by carefully modeling a more correct version, but they do not always demand perfection. The level of language proficiency that the parent requires gradually increases but remains flexible. The child's early attempts at communicating are successful largely because the listener mentally corrects and adds to what was said to form a whole thought (Dale, 1972). In this way a beginning vocabulary of a few words can communicate dozens of ideas between parent and child.

The process of learning to read and write is in real contrast to that of acquiring oral language. In the structured classroom setting with one or more adults, the beginning reader uses books with stories about experiences of other children—experiences visually impaired children may have missed. The words will approximate but not match their own language. The time and place for reading will be fairly consistent and have a clear beginning and ending. The child within a group will be directly instructed about "how to read." The best effort will usually be required and attempts at reading will be interpreted as either right or wrong.

AUDITORY DEVELOPMENT

A highly significant factor in readiness and success in early reading is skill in auditory discrimination. Auditory discrimination depends to a large extent on auditory acuity. Many visually impaired multihandicapped children, and especially deaf-blind children, because of losses in auditory acuity, will be unable to develop auditory discrimination or to detect likeness and difference among letter sounds as they occur in words. Losses in the high frequency ranges affect the child's ability to hear consonants such as "s," "t," "b," "p," "c," "u," and blends as "ch," "st," and "fl." Loss in the lower frequencies affects the child's ability to hear vowel sounds. Gleason (1984) in describing hearing losses in visually impaired children referred to conductive losses and sensorineural losses. Conductive losses are largely due to outer or middle ear injuries or infection and result in a general loss of volume. Sensorineural losses result from damage or deterioration of the inner ear or auditory nerve producing an inability to fully hear high frequency consonant sounds. Children with sensorineural or high frequency losses are at a real disadvantage since consonants carry most of the distinctive features of language necessary for comprehension.

For the child with normal hearing ability, learning to identify objects according to their sound is one step in auditory discrimination. Learning to identify mother by her voice or a rattle by its sound is an important first step. Learning to associate words with objects is an important next step in the sequence of learning to listen and to comprehend spoken language. A visually impaired child without other handicaps may develop quite readily in auditory discrimination. Since vision is not a distraction, the child may develop an excellent awareness of environmental sounds and notice differences in voices that fully sighted or partially sighted children may not notice. For a discussion of assessing listening skills and suggested teaching sequences and materials, see Chapter 9.

TACTUAL PERCEPTUAL DEVELOPMENT

The importance of visual acuity and visual perception to the reading success of sighted children has been greatly emphasized. Blind children need tactual readiness materials just as seeing children need visual reading readiness materials. The tactual discrimination of a braille cell requires a very special preliminary readiness program. A conclusion of the research by Nolan and Kederis (1969) indicated that braille word recognition was the result of the accumulation of information over a temporal interval. Integration of a sequence of touch sensations which are obtained when an individual handles an object is often called the haptic sense. Revesz (1950) concluded that totally blind people have the ability to perceive space haptically and that a necessary condition is movement of the body.

The American Printing House for the Blind has developed a variety of materials for use in developing the tactual readiness skills for the reading of braille dots. Tactual discrimination worksheets, puzzles, peg kits, formboards, and textured beads are among the many materials which are available (See Figure 4). A special program A Tactual Road to Reading, consists of a guidebook, lesson plans, and a series of tactual readiness books designed especially for children who will use braille as their reading medium (Kurzhals & Caton, 1974).

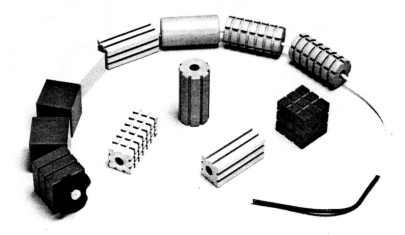

Figure 4. Giant Textured Beads, Courtesy of American Printing House for the Blind, Louisville, Kentucky.

In order to define touch sensitivity, Kurzhals (1966, 1974) recommended learning to distinguish objects which are alike from those which are different, and to use objects to teach size and shape discrimination. To acquire skill in the use of hands and fingers, she recommended having the child examine objects such as flowers, baby chickens, kittens, or small models of birds. To develop the skill of keeping the fingers moving rhythmically, she recommended having the child trace lines of yarn with the index finger of each hand. The patterns increased in difficulty as the child proceeded through a book of yarn-lined pages. The skill of moving the fingers from line to line down the page is developed through the use of a stick book. The child traced sticks of varying length across and down the page. Later, the child proceeded to a book with machine-sewn lines. To keep all the fingers of both hands curved comfortably on the page, she suggested having the child use its fingers to discriminate pages of cardboard geometric shapes. A book, *Touch and Tell* (see Figure 5) developed by the American Printing Houe for the Blind (Duncan, 1969), proceeds from embossed large hands and geometric shapes to smaller shapes and finally to braille lines and cells comparable to the dots found in beginning braille readers. Similar materials can be made by the teacher by using scrap felt materials, flocked paper, or scraps of materials.

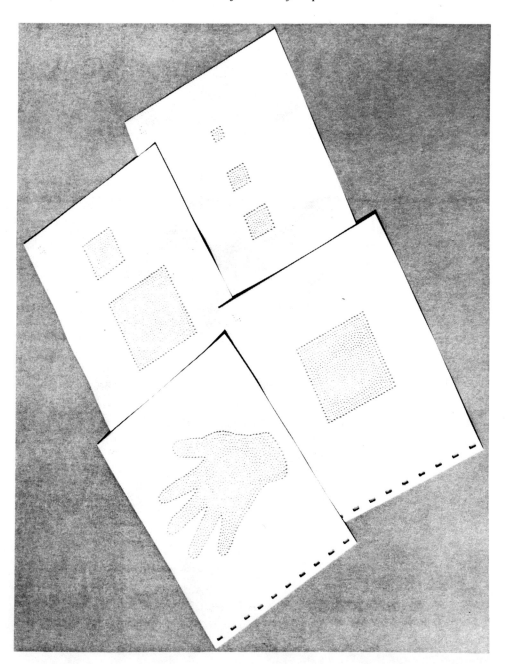

Figure 5. Pages from Touch and Tell.

The construction of teaching aids for teaching basic concepts of sensory development is described by Dorward and Barraga (1968) and Barraga, Dorward, and Ford (1973). Barraga (1976) has been very helpful in suggesting sequential lessons based on a developmental approach to tactual learning. This approach is helpful in that it provides a step-by-step sequence of activities which proceed from very gross tactual awareness to the very fine and precise skill of discrimintion and recognition of braille characters. These steps could be defined as:

1. Awareness of and attention to textures, temperatures, and other characteristics of three-dimensional objects
2. Discrimination of shape, size, weight, and later directional characteristics of objects so that three-dimensional objects can be recognized and labeled
3. Learning to recognize two-dimensional representations such as geometric shapes with the use of a variety of materials
4. Learning to discriminate and recognize braille characters

The most important principal in developing tactual readiness is to move from tactual discrimination of very gross patterns to tactual discrimination of very fine patterns (braille dots) through a series of small progressive sequential steps. The speed of progression should be varied according to the individual ability of each child.

Kershman (1976) validated an order of tactual discrimination tasks, using 60 young blind children. The following order was suggested:

1. Large solid geometric shapes
2. Flat (puzzle pieces) figures
3. Embossed dot geometric figures
4. Raised dot line figures
5. Braille letters

Young blind and low vision children should be encouraged to explore with their hands. Many tactually stimulating materials, such as common household items, are needed. Laura Bridgeman's favorite tactual object was her father's shoe. Commercial materials, such as the Tactual Stimulation Kit of the American Printing House for the Blind, can also be used for additional arousal of the child's tactual interests. Opportunities should be provided for finger manipulation in order to develop coordination and dexterity. Take-apart manipulative toys and puzzles could be used for developing this coordination. Texture and shape discrimination items will help readiness for learning to discriminate the fine differences in spatial relationships in dot configurations.

Millar (1978) found that exercises to process the dot pattern as a form rather than a set of dots would simplify the associative learning process. It was easier for the blind children to learn the tactual stimulus as an integrated shape rather than a set of complex inter-relationships of dots. The implication for the teacher is to use readiness materials of shape identification, such as *Touch and Tell* series from the American Printing House for the Blind rather than teaching the child dot patterns from memorization of dot numbers, such as the "p." The teacher may teach the child the shape and show how it differs from a shape like the "y." It is better, according to Millar (1975), to use contrasting shapes rather than similar shapes for encoding in memory. Similar shapes would cause more interference patterns with learning and would be more difficult to memorize. For example, "p" is similar to "f" or "v."

Mangold (1978) developed a program of tactile perception and braille letter recognition for use with braille readers. The program was used in a readiness program for beginning and remedial braille readers. The beginning readers using the program showed less scrubbing and backtracking behaviors and fewer errors in braille. The program was based on a precision teaching model with dot symbol tracking and identification exercises divided into 29 lessons.

MOTOR DEVELOPMENT

Young visually impaired children often need individual attention in muscular and motor development because of factors such as lack of sensory stimulation and complications from other physical disabilities. Buell (1966) found that over-protected and under-stimulated blind children perform far below the norms of other visually impaired children on gross motor activities such as running, jumping, and throwing.

Jankowski and Evans (1981) confirmed Buell's finding with 20 blind children who were characterized by "creeping overweight" with weak upper limbs and low aerobic capacity. Braille reading requires both perceptual and motor ability. Perception cannot occur except when the hands are moving across the braille symbols. The fingers of the hands must track from left-to-right across the line of braille and then make a return sweep to the next line.

Motor coordination is no less valued for the low vision student reading print who must align the book with the most acute vision in the better eye and coordinate neck and muscles to maintain best vision. Considerable concentration and attention is required for the low vision student to hold the book at the best focal distance and to maintain visual focus. The more limited the acuity the more difficult the physical aspects of the reading task.

Cutsforth (1951) recognized the danger of reading instruction with braille before the child had developed proper muscular maturation. He advocated activities such as running, jumping, wrestling, pounding, and sawing in developing the gross motor muscular system before moving into the fine motor activities such as braille and large print reading and writing. A good readiness program for braille reading would require fine motor hand coordination. An example of recognizing the need for this type of fine motor coordination was the sewing outline cards taken by Ann Sullivan Macy to Tecumseh to begin instruction with Helen Keller. Suggestions for fine motor coordination activities can be found in *Reach Out and Teach* (Ferrell, 1985). The ability to use one's fingers well, as is necessary for braille reading, is helped through practice. "This entails first doing things with the whole body, then with the arms and hands and large muscles, and later doing fine things which strengthen the fingers and make them more flexible and sensitive" (Halliday, 1970, p. 65).

Perceptual-motor "body image" development is an important component of a reading readiness program. Body image may be defined as "a knowledge of body parts, how the parts relate to each other, how the parts may be utilized both individually and collectively for purposeful activity, and how the parts relate to the child's spatial environment" (Mills, 1970, p. 81). Important aspects of body image development for blind children identified by Cratty and Sams (1968) include body planes, parts and movements, and left-right discrimination. A body image test was developed to assess these and other more complex body image areas. Examples of related activities include the following:

- Simon Says
- Rhythmic activities
- Skipping rope
- Creeping and walking obstacle courses
- Stepping games
- Jointed doll movements

Hill (1986) suggested an integrative concept development program in which the teacher of the visually impaired would coordinate the teaching of needed concepts throughout the child's school program. For example, concepts such a "up," "down," "under," "above," could be taught during transition activities. "Put your book *under* the desk." "Stand *up* if you can hear me," etc. Assessment of such concepts could be obtained through the Hill Performance Test of Selected Positional Concepts (Hill, 1981). The teacher could develop a list of these important concepts on reading readiness and assist the regular classroom teacher in integrating them within her overall program.

EMOTIONAL AND SOCIAL DEVELOPMENT

Emotional stability has an important effect upon reading success. Many visually impaired children come to school with emotional problems fostered at home by parents who are overprotective or rejective. Sommers (1944), using the California Personality Test and interviews with parents, found five patterns of parental reaction to their blind children: (1) acceptance, (2) denial, (3) over-protectiveness, (4) overt rejection, and (5) disguised rejection. Their children exhibited six patterns of adjustive reaction which were closely related to the parental reactions. Teachers may help to insure emotional success in beginning reading by several means:

1. The teacher should provide an atmosphere of acceptance by loving and respecting the individual personality of each child.
2. The teacher should behave in an emotionally mature manner.
3. An atmosphere of calm, courtesy, and happiness should prevail in the classroom.
4. Directions and suggestions should be positive, and praise should be used liberally as a reward for appropriate behavior.
5. Self-confidence should be nourished by carefully leading each child through an individualized readiness program with sequential steps which are small enough to be readily accomplished.
6. Simple routines should be established in the classroom so that each child knows what is expected and what activities can be expected during the day. Periods of freedom to play and to enjoy large-muscle activities should be regular and frequent.
7. Braille reading should be postponed for some children until they are emotionally ready to begin. Listening skills are especially important to visually impaired children, and listening can be the focus of learning for the child not ready to begin reading. Many visually impaired children may need an extra year or more in a readiness program before starting into a reading program. Some visually impaired children, especially those who are multihandicapped, may not profit

from a braille reading program. Premature exposure to reading may frustrate the child and cause a serious setback to self-confidence and positive self-image.

Many visually impaired children have had little, if any, contact with peer groups of children before entering school. Their interaction with other children may be egocentric. Limited vision deprives them of an important means of evaluating the reactions of others to their action.

Limited vision imposes a special handicap on participation in game-like activities with other children. The visually impaired child is somewhat limited in awareness of what is going on during the game and the attitudes of the other players. The low vision child may have a better idea but is still at considerable disadvantage. The child must depend on sound localization, voice identification, and physical contact and perhaps some visual information as basic sources of information. It becomes very difficult to form a concept of the game and the relationship of the players and to compete successfully with little or no vision.

INTELLECTUAL DEVELOPMENT

Traditionally, children are supposed to be "ready" to read when they obtain a mental age of six and one-half years (Dolch, 1950). Lowenfeld, Abel, and Hatlen (1969) found a very high correlation between intelligence and reading ability in visually impaired readers. Since intelligence tests are largely made up of items requiring verbal comprehension and language ability, measured intelligence could be a determining factor in reading success, especially if the mesurement deviates far from the average.

Some educators feel that too much emphasis is placed on braille reading for children of low intelligence. For instance, Nolan and Kederis (1969) assert that for children with intelligence quotients below 85, braille is an extremely inefficient medium of communication. On the other hand, some basic braille reading skills may be taught very successfully to some low functioning children. Even a low level of Grade 1 braille reading ability may be very helpful in daily living skills as reading labels on canned goods, clothing, colors, the numbers on a watch, or telephone numbers.

ORIENTATION TO BOOKS

The normally sighted child generally enters school with a knowledge of books from experience looking at pictures in magazines and picture story books. Many visually impaired children lack experience in the handling of books. Kurzhals (1966) suggests that the child be given books of different sizes and shapes to examine. These books can be made by the teacher with heavy cardboard and fastened together with steel rings. The books can be made interesting to the child by placing different textures and shapes of materials on each page to explore.

Visually impaired children need to gain experience in orienting the book in a comfortable position and in turning the pages from left to right. They also need to learn simple concepts which will be useful in following the reading directions of the teacher such as top, bottom, right, and left, as related to the sides of the book. They may be asked to locate specific shapes or textures which are attached at various positions on each page. As the children proceed through the book, the pages become a little more complex with the addition of other shapes or textures.

In order to develop the necessary mechanics without too much repetition with the same books, the teacher can develop a number of different kinds of tactual books. Kurzhals (1974) in Tactual Road to Reading describes several kinds of tactual books which give variety to the program:

1. A cloth book with an envelope on the cover filled with different pieces of cloth to match with cloth on each page of the book.
2. A paper book with scratchy, bumpy silky, smooth, and rough paper to examine.
3. A flower book with a different shaped flower made from chenille, pipestem cleaners, or wood fiber (scrap felt paper from the florist or scrap wallpaper samples could be used in this book).
4. A button book with many different shaped buttons arranged in a variety of ways on each page.
5. A zipper book with pockets containing small toys and objects to identify.
6. An envelope book with each page having an envelope containing an object representing a word with a different sound.

The following checklist may help to evaluate "book behavior" of young visually impaired children. Before beginning reading, each child should have had certain experiences with books.

- The child feels secure with books and likes to play with and handle books.
- The child shows respect for books by taking care of them.
- The child locates the front, back, top, and bottom of the book.
- The child turns the pages in consecutive order.
- The child uses hands or eyes in a left-right movement to follow a line across the page.
- The child listens attentively to stories read from a book.
- The child remembers and relates the stories in the book.
- The child locates the spatial positions on the page: up, down, left, and right.
- The child uses hands or eyes successfully in the return sweep from right to left to locate the next line on the page.

MOBILITY

The mobility skills of young blind children are extremely important in enabling them to move about in their environments to obtain concrete experience. These concrete experiences are necessary to build the concepts and language which will make reading meaningful and motivating. Mobility can be enhanced through sensory training and the development of basic concepts and motor skills and precane mobility skills.

A project (Harley, Wood, and Merbler, 1975) was conducted in orientation and mobility for multiply impaired blind children who were functioning on a preschool level. The objectives of this project were to develop, to refine, and to validate programmed instruction in orientation and mobility for use by classroom teachers and parents. Lessons were programmed in small sequential steps with directions to the teacher or parent showing when to give commands, reinforce, repeat cycles, or proceed to the next step. The programmed instruction was divided into four categories: (1) motor development, (2) sensory skills, (3) concept development, and (4) mobility skills. The motor section was divided into nine sections proceeding from basic movement and creeping to jumping and climbing. Sensory training included sound localization and tactual and olfactory discrimination. Concept development skills ranged from simple body image and size-shape discriminations to the spatial relations concepts of front-back, up-down, and left-right. The mobility skills consisted of specialized techniques such as trailing, use of sighted guide, and utilization of discriminable landmarks. The results of the research indicated significantly higher scores for the experimental over the control group, and validated the programmed instruction for use with other multihandicapped blind children. This program was extended to include visually   impaired infants and toddlers in the areas of motor, cognitive, auditory and tactual perception (Harley & Long, 1986).

MOTIVATION

Reading can be very exciting, and the teacher can help to make it that way. Miller (1985) described readiness experiences with her own blind child with suggestions for adapting print books for preschool blind children. She listed appropriate commercially produced books with tactual adaptations, such as Golden Book's Touch and Feel series and What's That? by Philomel Books. She also described ways to make reading more motivating for visually impaired children such as:

1. Making tactual pictures such as using "fur" to represent a dog, "beans" on cover of Jack and the Beanstalk, etc.
2. Letting the child turn pages as mother reads the story.
3. Leaving words off of the ends of sentences for the listening child to fill in the blanks only.
4. Making book bags, placing the book in a bag with objects mentioned in the story.
5. Having family members act out the story using real objects such as ladder, laundry basket, handcuffs, etc.
6. Tracking braille or print sentences rather than using readiness book materials.
7. Using commercial story books with tactual pictures.

Computer graphics programs that allow a braille printer to produce pictures, graphs, and maps are available and should increase the availability of graphics to braille students. The teacher can make reading motivating to visually impaired children by becoming excited and involved with the story. The stories can be made more meaningful by having the child experience the concepts in the stories through bringing in objects to the classroom and taking the children on field trips. Stories may be dramatized. Instructional materials with bright colors and exciting textures and sounds may be used. For example, one teacher made a "mouse book" of readiness materials with embossed lines on the pages for the children to trace. As they trace the lines, the teacher would tell the story of a mouse. At the end of one line the mouse found some cheese, and at the end of another line a cat, etc. This booklet of tactual readiness exercises contained a life-size rubber mouse attached to the book that could be handled and squeezed to make mouse-type noises. This exercise was exciting, and meaningful, and fun.

SUMMARY

The teacher of beginning braille or print reading may carefully develop a reading readiness program which considers each of the preceding factors. However, it should be emphasized that a child's desire to read underlies the total readiness program. Some visually impaired children may have developed a desire to read through observation of parents and siblings at home. Helen Keller developed a curiosity for reading through observing her father read a newspaper. Visually impaired children are restricted through limited vision from observing many opportunities for incidental reading which occurs through signs on the streets, labels on foodstuffs, or advertisements on television. In many homes, sighted children often observe the reading activities of family members. They delight in having a family member read to them and share the excitement of a fascinating or favorite story. They learn to explore magazines and picture books long before they enter school.

Visually impaired children usually need additional and special experiences in handling tactile or large print books in order to develop meaningful attitudes toward reading. Reading aloud to them from print books is especially important in developing a desire to read. However, the children need to experience and enjoy the concepts represented in the stories contained in the words and pictures.

Visually impaired children who have brothers and sisters in school may be stimulated to want to read if their siblings have developed healthy attitudes toward reading. Building a desire to read may require a considerable period of time for some children. Beginning reading instruction before fostering a desire to read may cause a negative and damaging attitude which could insure reading failure from the start. Leading the child into reading by developing a classroom environment which makes the child feel secure and which stimulates the child to desire to read is more likely to insure a successful beginning.

CHAPTER 3

APPROACHES TO READING INSTRUCTION

THE VISION specialist's best preparation for teaching reading to visually impaired students is a thorough knowledge of the effective approaches and alternative materials for teaching reading to normally sighted students. The vision teacher will need to combine a variety of methodologies to meet the unique learning strengths and needs of visually impaired children who are learning to read through print, enlarged print, or braille.

The purpose of this chapter is not to discuss in detail the various methods for teaching reading. There are many excellent texts that serve this purpose (Aulls, 1982). However, a survey of current approaches as they relate to visually impaired students using print, large print, or braille should be helpful. Three methods to teaching reading are presented: whole word, phonic, and linguistic. A "method" is defined by the authors as the major strategy that the student is taught to use to identify words. All three methods are components of the best approach. These methods are followed by four formats for organizing the reading materials: basal reader, individualized format, programmed materials, and language experience format. The effectiveness of the format seems to be dependent on the attitude of the teacher using the format. If the teacher believes in the format, it will most likely be effective (Bond & Dykstra, 1967).

A format, such as a basal reader, may provide instruction in each method of word identification with early emphasis on one method, such as the recognition of whole words. The method and the format together constitute an approach to reading.

An effective combination of methods and formats that become an approach to teaching reading will vary depending on whether the reading medium is large print or braille. However, the methods and formats for teaching reading through braille or large print have more commonalities than differences (see Figure 6).

39

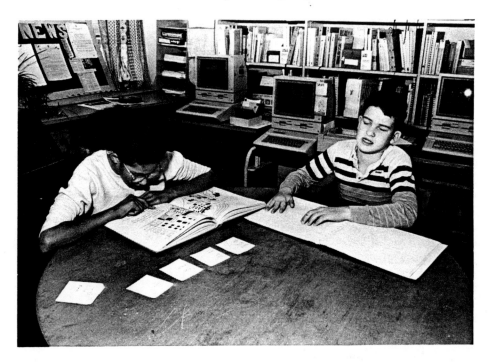

Figure 6. Teaching reading through print or braille has more commonalities than differences.

The processes of braille and print reading are essentially the same in three vital components. First, the ultimate goal of communicating ideas is identical whether the individual uses embossed dots, ink print, or some other medium for reading. Second, regardless of the medium, the process of reading involves an abstraction of personal experiences. There is no meaning on the printed page, only ink; there is no meaning on the braille page, only dots. In each instance the meaning is in the mind of the reader. The reader brings meaning to the page from the store of experiences. Whether the child is blind or sighted, the background of experience is the core of reading. For the child who is visually impaired, this core of experience may be comparatively limited in scope, breadth, and depth. This limitation must receive primary attention during the readiness program and throughout reading instruction.

The third component of reading that is common regardless of the medium employed is the interaction that takes place within the brain. New experiences, new meanings, and new ideas instantly interact, expanding and/or modifying those concepts previously stored in the mind. Thus, the comprehension skills involving the various cognitive processes will be constant in both visual and tactual reading. The visually impaired children who are learning to read are not learning to read large print or braille. They are learning to read, and they are learning through the medium of enlarged print or braille.

The methods and formats that make up approaches to reading instruction discussed in this chapter are targeted for beginning and early reading instruction. Alternative approaches for remedial reading instruction will be discussed in Chapter 7. Methods and formats for teaching students who need to learn braille after acquiring beginning reading proficiency will be discussed in Chapter 10. The three methods by which the reader may identify words (whole word, phonic, and linguistic) are alternative methods. Each has an appropriate context and all are necessary for efficient reading.

A continuing controversy has ensued among educators and publishers of books for normally sighted students as to the relative merits of the phonetic or synthetic method and the whole-word or analytic method of reading instruciton. Jeanne Chall's very popular book, *Learning to Read: The Great Debate* (1967) enumerates the many shifts in emphasis since the beginning of public instruction in this country. The linguistic method, which developed in the past 30 years, is now embroiled in the controversy of methodology. Each method is necessary for well-rounded word identification skill. One method alone may help some children learn to read well. On the other hand, reliance on one method also produces some unsuccessful readers. Research can be cited to support each method, yet, too frequently research involves such a large number of variables that interpretation becomes difficult.

METHODS OF TEACHING READING

Whole-Word Method

Using a whole-word method, children are first taught to recognize words and phrases as distinctive for the overall shape, length, or unique features of the word. The crucial element is quickly and accurately identifying words by associating the total meaning with the symbolic representation. Whole word methodology is based on the premise that reading is more than identifying words; it also emphasizes acquring meaning. The most effective way to teach words is not through letter sounds but through the uniqueness of each word. Such a premise labels phonetics, or any form of direct sound-symbol instruction, as mechanical and distracting to the acquisition of meaning.

A format that emphasizes a whole-word method in beginning reading relies on structuring the order of introduction of words and the repetition rate of words within the book. Frequency count studies of the most common words are the basis of the order of introduction of words with the most frequently used words occurring earlier in the series.

In the beginning of instruction the goal is to help the child develop a basic reading vocabulary that is recognized "on sight." This basic reading vocabulary is expanded as the child encounters words of increasing similarity requiring the child to refine methods of recognition and move beyond overall shape to beginning and ending letter and unusual letter sequences.

The child who has developed a basic sight vocabulary, i.e., words that were recognized instantly as wholes, is guided in the beginning to analyze those same words. The assumption is that if children can analyze the component sounds of words that they can already read they will be able to use the same strategy to attack unfamiliar words. In a strictly whole-word method, much of this discovery, or analytic process, is only an incidental part of the reading program; there is little sequential development of word attack skills. Some children become very successful in reading by means of the whole-word method. Others fail to develop a sufficient skill in attacking new words to become good independent readers. Studies of the compatibility between reading with large print and a whole-word method were not found in the literature. However, the relationship between reading with braille and a whole-word method has been examined in several studies (Kusajima, 1974; Lowenfeld, Abel, & Hatlen, 1969; Nolan & Kederis, 1969).

During the early 50s when there was a strong emphasis upon the whole-word method of reading instruction, leaders in the area of the education of the blind began advocating the introduction of Grade 2 braille, with its many contracted forms, in the initial stages of instruction. Prior to this time, when braille was first officially adopted in this country, beginning readers were taught to read in full spelling, known as Grade 1 braille. Later, 45 contractions were added to shorten the amount of space required for the code, and beginning reading materials were embossed in this form, known as Grade 1-1/2. The more highly contracted form, Grade 2, was not introduced until near the end of the elementary grades. Whether or not the popularity of the whole-word method exerted any causal effect upon the shift to the use of the highly contracted, shortened braille orthography in beginning reading materials, the time relationship is interesting.

Methods of teaching braille reading can be classified according to two dimensions: analytic or synthetic approach, and the degree of structure in the reading materials. Much of the research has been concerned with the analytic versus the synthetic approaches to the teaching of braille reading. In an early book on teaching braille reading, Maxfield (1928) noted that the majority of teachers of blind children favored the whole-word system. In a teacher survey, she found three methods of teaching reading: (1) the letter method, (2) the word method, and (3) the letter-word method. Maxfield recommended that the word method was the most reliable method in the teaching of reading to braille readers, and that blind children should obtain a touch vocabulary of at least 200 words before learning to put words together by sound.

Lowenfeld, Abel, and Hatlen (1969) authored the first American book on the teaching of reading to blind children after the one by Katherine Maxfield in 1928. *Blind Children Learn to Read* was oriented primarily around a study by the authors on the teaching of braille reading to blind children. Their study had the purpose of describing the status of braille reading to blind children and instruction in local schools and residential schools for the blind. It also had the purpose of determining the characteristics and the reading behavior of efficient and inefficient braille readers. In the first part of the study, questionnaires were returned from teachers in 289 local and 73 residential schools. Two-thirds of the teachers used the braille alphabet. All of the readers with few exceptions started with Grade 2 braille. A major finding from this study was that most teachers in day schools and residential schools used the whole-word method in the teaching of beginning reading to blind chldren.

Kusajima (1974) studied the physiology and psychology of tactual and visual reading in a series of studies which took place over a period of 35 years. The original Japanese edition, which was published in 1969, was finally translated into English and published in 1974. Kusajima studied blind and partially seeing students who read braille using an apparatus consisting of a tactual recorder. This tactual recorder was composed of a ring on the finger with an arm which extended out over the fingers. A stylus was attached to the arm which marked a recording drum. As the braille reader moved the fingers across the material, the drum moved at the same time. The result was a visual record of finger movements. The material given to the students varied from short, easy-to-read sentences of three to four lines in length to foreign words and nonsense words of braille letters. Groups of subjects ranged in size from 12 to 164 boys and girls; ages ranged from 10 to 23.

Kusajima concluded that braille characters are perceived successfully through movement of the fingers. Among the best readers, letters become grouped in perception as words or short sentences as in visual reading. He based his theory of Gestalt reading on the basis of movement of the fingers. Up and down movements indicated letter-by-letter reading, whereas smooth, horizontal lines indicated Gestalt reading. Uneven pressure indicated letter-by-letter or symbol-by-symbol reading, and even pressure indicated perception of whole words and sentences.

Although conceding that braille characters were at first perceived successively through movement of the fingers, he felt that a group of braille cells might later be perceived as a totality, or gestalt, as words or short sentences. A distinction was made between good and poor readers; the good readers perceived a gestalt of words or short sentences, but the poor readers perceived each character one-at-a-time in a letter-by-letter method.

Kusajima, discounted the theory of two-handed braille reading in which one hand takes on the function of synthesis, while the other takes on the function of analysis of braille characters. He showed that hand movements were uniform in rate and parallel in displacement, demonstrating the insignificant difference in reading performance between reading with one hand as compared with reading with two hands. He concluded that in the two-handed reading of braille texts, one finger reads while the other checks and confirms what has been read.

Kusajima determined that visual and tactual reading were identical except that the pause of the eye in visual reading was equivalent to movement of the fingers in braille reading. He conceded that characters were perceived successfully, and that the unit of perception was not as wide as in visual reading. However, braille reading speeds were not as slow as one would predict on the basis of number of perceptual units because perception was combined with other functions such as use of context. The greater the reader's experience, intelligence, and understanding of the text, the fewer were the unnecessary hand movements in reading the braille text. He finally concluded that a row of homogeneous figures was both differentiated and integrated at the same time. Therefore, in tactile reading, comprehension occurred through appreciation of whole-word and whole-sentence configurations (not through the

·integration of individual letters), and through cognitive linking of sentence meanings.

Support for the whole-word approach can be found in more recent research. Pring (1985) concluded, after comparing 10 blind children and five blind adults with 18 sighted children with similar comprehension levels, the blind students do not construct a phonological letter-by-letter code in identifying pseudohomophones, such as "BLOO" or "BRANE." This finding may have been due to their need for allocation of more attention to feature analysis and perceptual processes leaving less time for phonological analysis, or it may be due to the low redundancy of the braille code compared to print. The results from this study might also suggest use of a whole-word approach in identification of words by these blind children and adults. This study may have obtained different results had the blind and sighted subjects been more comparable in chronological age in addition to reading comprehension.

The continued popularity of the whole-word method among teachers of the visually impaired was found in a survey of residential schools for the blind (LaSasso & Jones, 1984). The results indicated that the most used basal reader was the Ginn 720 series (41%). The Patterns series was the next most used series by 31% of the schools, whereas, Basics in Reading (28%) and the Ginn 360 series (11%) were the most used reading series. Both Ginn basal readers stressed a whole-word method to reading.

Phonetic Method

During the first decade of this century, a strong emphasis was placed on the phonetic method for teaching reading to normally sighted students (Chall, 1967). Throughout the shifting popularity of the phonetic method, the readers were taught to associate sounds instead of mere letter names with the symbols. The students then blended, or synthesized those sounds to identify words. Advocates pointed out that since the symbol functions within a word, not by virtue of name but by virtue of the sound that it represents, word recognition would thus be facilitated (Fries, 1963). Proponents claim that the readers soon gained skill and independence in sounding out new words.

Critics find several weaknesses in this phonetic, or synthetic, approach to reading (Gates, 1922). The initial processes may be slow and void of meaning, causing many children to lose interest in reading. Students might become word-callers instead of searchers for meaning.

One of the greatest difficulties in the phonetics approach is the fact that our language is not highly consistent in its sound-spelling patterns. Spache and Spache (1973) concluded that relatively few phonic rules have a high degree of usefulness. They recommended that teachers teach students to look for probabilities for word pronunciation using these specific rules and not focus on confusing discrepancies of the phonic rules.

It may be argued that phonetic rules have a fairly low degree of reliability and that their use is frequently in reverse to that of the reading process. For example, although the reading sweep is from left to right, many vowel sounds are controlled by an element such as the "r" or silent "e" which follows rather than precedes them. Since the unit of tactual perception and low vision perception is much smaller than the unit of normal visual perception, visually impaired children cannot easily look ahead to facilitate the application of those cues. The most successful approaches include instruction in letter/sound relationships or phonetics. Chall (1967) summarizing research on phonetic methods of reading instruction concluded, "Progress may be slower with a phonic emphasis than with other approaches, but the end results are probably more satisfactory." (p. 177).

Nolan and Kederis (1969) attempted to determine the perceptual factors in braille word recognition through a series of nine experiments. Using the tachistotactometer, a device for exposing braille cells and words for controlled periods of time, they found that:

1. character recognition time was related to the number of dots within a character, the spread of dots within a group of characters, the location of dots in the upper or lower part of the cell, and their frequency of occurrence in print;
2. the exposure time for word recognition was longer than the sums of the recognition times for the individual braille characters which made up each word;
3. recognition times for braille words became greater with decrease in familiarity, inclusion of contractions, increase in length, and shift in dot distributions from concentrations in the upper parts of the braille cell;
4. peripheral cues derived from preceding context, experience with the probabilities with which letters and letter groups follow one another in print, and knowledge of the grammatical properties of the language played a part in word recognition time.

The results of this research by Nolan and Kederis (1969) indicated that whole-word reading was not characteristic of braille readers, and that the perceptual unit in word recognition was the braille cell. The principal evidence for this conclusion resulted from the finding that the recognition of braille words required from 16 to 196% more time than the sums of the times required to recognize the individual characters. Supportive evidence for this conclusion was drawn from the results which show that training in character recognition can result in significant increases in accuracy of silent reading, increased speed of oral reading, and decreased errors in oral reading for elementary grade braille readers. Nolan and Kederis (1969) concluded that word recognition appeared to be a sequential integrative process, one in which word recognition is the result of the accumulation of information over a temporal interval. They suggested that the probability of letter sequences and contextual clues could help the reader identify a word correctly before all of its characters were touched.

Among the recommendations made by Nolan and Kederis (1969) in the teaching of braille reading were:

1. Stress tactual perceptual development in the preschool and primary years, starting with gross examination of real objects and proceeding through stages to a final stage stressing braille character recognition.
2. Emphasize character recognition in the early stages of reading instruction.
3. Maintain constant monitoring of character recognition skills.

The careful reader will note the quite different conclusions derived by the research of Nolan and Kederis (1969) and Kusajima (1974). Nolan and Kederis concluded that the cell is the unit of perception in braille reading while Kusajima concluded that groups of braille characters were perceived as a whole. The differences in the populations and methodologies probably influence the different conclusions and limit comparison of the studies. In comparing populations it can be observed that Kasajima's subjects were largely adults and included many fluent and experienced braille readers. Nolan and Kederis' subjects were elementary and high school students and included a wide range of proficiency levels. In methodology Kusajima used a rolling drum and ring for monitoring reading behavior. Nolan and Kederis used a tachistotachometer and time samples of individual character recognition and recognition of words.

A careful comparison of the two studies may reveal that the two conclusions may not be as different as it first appears. Kusajima, Clark, and

Jastrembska found character-by-character reading in poor readers and found that reading by words and phrases required greater intelligence and experience. He also found that even the best readers read cell-by-cell when analyzing unfamiliar words. The importance of context found by Kusajima, Clark, and Jastrembska suggests the importance of a third method of word identification: the linguistics method.

Linguistic Method

Within recent years, the linguistics theory has been having an impact on the field of reading instruction. Goodman (1973), defined it as the scientific study and analysis of language. Linguists analyze language under three domains: (1) phonology, the sound-spelling or phoneme-grapheme relationship, (2) syntax or structural grammar, and (3) semantics or meaning. Reading which is a language process, and linguistics, which is the science of language, should be closely allied. Although not an approach in itself, linguistics theory, if correctly applied, adds a third method to reading instruction.

Bloomfield and Barnhart (1961) and Fries (1963) were among the first linguists to apply linguistic theory to reading instruction. They emphasized the phonological characteristics of language. American English has been identified to have 46 phonemes which are the smallest significant units of sound. But some of these sounds have several spelling patterns. Hanna, Hodges, and Hanna (1971) found that a computer programmed with spelling rules could spell 50% of the 17,000 most common English words.

Bloomfield and Barnhart (1961), Fries (1963), Spache and Spache (1973) stressed the systematic introduction of only the regular sound-spelling units during the initial stages of reading. They advocated the introduction of the most common whole words while simultaneously guiding children to discover the significant contrasting elements between words, thus developing the concept of the phoneme-morpheme-grapheme relationship. They stressed that, since the meaning is already couched in the oral language, reading becomes a decoding process to discover sound relationships.

Current linguists and psycholinguists, such as Goodman (1973) and Smith (1978), place strong emphasis upon the element of meaning as the essential core of reading, and on the interaction or co-action of phonetic, syntactic, and semantic cues in supplying that meaning. Smith defined "information" as the reduction of uncertainty and described these three cues as "redundant" or overlapping in providing information for reduction of uncertainty. For example, within words there are certain spelling probabilities; within sentences certain syntactical probabilities; and within context certain meaning probabilities, all of which are cues to limit the possible alternatives or uncertainties about a given word. The skilled, fluent reader depends much more highly upon syntactic and semantic cues than upon the spelling pattern. When the analysis of an unknown visual or tactual spelling pattern becomes necessary, Smith would approach the process by word analogy or synonym.

Smith's discussion of information as the reduction of uncertainty is interesting if the ideas are applied to reading braille. He employs the illustration of the child who, looking at a print letter, has 26 possible alternatives for identifying that letter. These uncertainties must be reduced to one. An application of that illustration to the child reading braille suggests some startling comparisons. The child has under the fingers one perceptual unit: the cell. This unit represents 63 alternatives because there are 63 possible dot combinations. But many of those dot combinations represent more than one meaning. A rough tabulation of those additional meanings adds 72 more alternatives for a possible 135 possibilities in the literary code. Since these same configurations have additional meanings in the braille codes for mathematics and music, the number of possible alternatives is staggering. Therefore, the braille reader needs to learn to make optimal use of every semantic and syntatic cue available.

This discussion of linguistics theory and the presentation of the various linguistic methods of reading instruction are an overview of some significant aspects as applied to readers of braille or large print. For a more thorough background, the reader should refer to the references and to other textbooks on the method in question.

ORGANIZATIONAL FORMATS

Basal Reader Format

Basal reading series are used by a majority of schools as the core of the reading program. This statement also holds true for instruction in large print or braille. A basal reading series may combine elements of the whole-word, phonics, and linguistics methods in word identification. Basal readers are designed as sequenced instructional programs.

Most series begin with readiness material and move through two to four preprimers, one or two primers, and reading books of gradually increasing difficulty and interest up through the sixth or eighth grade. Books may be designated by level and or by grades. Accompanying workbooks or worksheets are usually designed to provide additional practice on specific reading skills and to integrate writing. The basal reading series is designated to consider the child's developmental readiness in the introduction of new skills. Many series include a total language package with spelling, English, handwriting, and listening components. Some series have upper, middle, and lower difficulty strands, parallel library books, duplicating masters, word cards, accompanying audiovisual aids, and computer software. Teacher guides offer many excellent suggestions from which teachers may select learning activities. Most include a reproduction of the student text with suggested comprehension questions, answers and vocabulary drills.

The reading vocabulary during the early levels is controlled for difficulty, rate of introduction, and sufficient repetition for mastery by most students. The vocabulary at the preprimer levels is supplemented by attractive pictures to give meaning to the words and to carry a meaningful plot to the story. In some series, rebus pictures are used within the text to represent special words that add variety to the story, but the picture words are not intended for mastery. Practice with skills for word mastery, word attack, and comprehension are presented throughout the series.

The majority of basal series control the story content in an effort to provide a proportional representation of different ethnic groups, various cultural backgrounds, and socioeconomic levels. Sex differences are considered so that girls may be heroines as frequently as boys are heroes. Publishers present a variety of illustration styles ranging from photographs to cartoons. Print changes in style, size, and intensity. Content of passages foster a variety of reading purposes, including reading directions, maps, graphs, charts, tables, plays, advertisements, poetry, fiction, and content areas of science and social studies.

Visually imparied readers may face possible pitfalls in the use of basal reader formats. Even with a wealth and variety of basal materials, the teacher must be ambitious and creative to adapt the instruction for the unique needs of each visually impaired reader. If the teacher fails to be diagnostic and selective in the use of methods and materials, some students will be bored, wasting precious learning time on busy work, and others will be frustrated, not being able to keep pace with the basal approach. Sheldon (1969) suggested that in a regular first grade class of 30 children, two can probably skip the readiness skills and complete the entire program in a few months; eight can skip the readiness training and complete the program by the end of the year; 15 will need all of the readiness materials but will complete the entire program by the end of the year; five will spend the entire year struggling through the readiness and preprimer phases of the program. A typical seventh grade class contains students with reading abilities ranging from grades 3 to 11 and a typical fourth grade ranges from 1 to 8. The teacher must be able to diagnose the individual needs and select and adapt materials to meet this wide range of learning styles and levels of ability.

For a student who is visually impaired, the basal reader contains some additional limitations to challenge the creativity of the teacher. In the process of transcribing the materials into braille or photoenlarging into large print, much of the meaning and motivation so carefully built in through the attractive pictures is deleted. The words of a preprimer may have little meaning when they stand alone. The teacher must use ingenuity to compensate for the absence of the picture in braille and the absence of color in the pictures in large print. An immediate help for the low vision print reader is for the teacher to make available a regular print copy of the student's book that has the colored pictures. Even students who read braille may gain some information through the colored pictures. Another possible way to interpret the meaning in pictures for blind readers is to have sighted classmates describe the pictures. This procedure is of questionable value because at a time when it is of utmost importance to strengthen the self-concept of the blind child by providing successful experiences, the blind students are constantly being reminded that sighted peers have better access to some forms of information in their basal readers.

A more positive method of supplying meaning without pictures may be dramatization prior to the reading of the story. The actors may be the children or dolls or puppets that the children manipulate. Another possible interpretation is for the teacher to supply the meaning and excitement of the plot, not by describing pictures, but by telling the story in an exciting way. In the telling, the teacher can lead up to each point at which the words of the book may be incorporated into the story and then allow the children to read those words. Thus, the children participate in the story themselves. As a review of the reading and an aid to comprehension skills, the teacher may later ask the children to read the words from the book and tell why certain characters talked or acted as they did.

Teachers may plan to introduce the vocabulary in informal classroom learning activities prior to any use of the book. Upon encountering the same words in the book, the student will have a better chance of reading with reasonable fluency.

Stories in the basal reader may be based on experiences not yet encountered by the young visually impaired child. Teachers must become familiar with the stories the child will be meeting through the series so that they can provide the essential background of experience through such channels as play, dramatization, and field trips. Occasionally, stories are so visual that the key experience cannot be understood by the child who is blind. The vision teacher may create an alternative story line to fit the dialogue and narrative of the story.

For the braille student, one problem associated with most commercially available basal reading programs is that they are sequential in terms of the print code. The orthography of braille is such that the relative word difficulty is not comparable in the two codes. The difficulty of the vocabulary in the early reading materials is increased for the braille reader because embossed words appear in varying forms under varying circumstances. For example, eight common service words: enough, his, in, was, were, to, into, and by, known as the lower whole-word signs, found in beginning materials have two entirely different forms according to the position within the sentence. Thus, for the braille reader, each becomes the equivalent of two words instead of one. In planning early reading materials for the print reader, publishers frequently state that inflections or words with new endings such as "ing" or "es," are not considered as new words. Therefore, authors do not have to plan for the frequency of repetition that would be necessary for mastery of a new word. In the braille code, many inflections are "new words" for the beginning reader; for example, the reader sees only the letter "l" as the form for "like." However, when "likes" is presented, that word must be in full spelling. The student's recognition process is not the mere addition of an "s" to an already known root word. Other factors related to the development of word attack skills will be discussed more fully in Chapter 4.

Currently, the American Printing House for the Blind produces a basal reading series, PATTERNS, which covers readiness through third grade levels, and is written especially for the braille reader. The content is selected to be meaningful to the visually impaired child. Introduction of vocabulary and word attack skills is sequenced on the basis of braille difficulty. This effort was a "first" in the production of braille reading materials in the specialists from several areas focused their attention upon the needs of the braille reader. The series was written by an editor in the area of reading textbooks for sighted children. The advisory committee included a linguist who supervised the sequencing of braille contractions and phonological patterns and experienced teachers of reading to visually impaired children.

In selecting an approach of teaching reading, the teacher of visually impaired students must weigh the relative merits of the various formats with the needs and skills of the individual student. Basal readers have the advantage of having a built-in gradually introduced vocabulary based on the most frequently occurring words (Fry, 1972). The order of vocabulary introduction is fairly consistent across publishers so that a student who can read 3^1 (first half of the third grade) book in one series may read a book graded for the same level in another series. Basals may integrate the language arts curriculum of reading, spelling, writing, and listening through booster activities such as games, manipulative materials, read-along books and records, charts, and films. Publishers may provide supplemental books that match the vocabulary of the basal reader to provide additional reading practice. These books may parallel the basal or may be remedial or enrichment readers.

A basal reader may have disadvantages for use with a particular child if the introduction of new vocabulary is too rapid and there is too little repetition of new words. Materials identified by the publisher as "supplemental" may actually be only tangentially related to the presentation of vocabulary in the reader. The readability level or grade level difficulty of the basal reader may be difficult to identify. The vision specialist may refer to the American Printing House for the Blind catalogues of braille and large print publications for a quick reference to the publisher's estimate of the reading level.

Individualized Format

An individualized format makes use of any available reading material that interest the particular student. The most common sources of materials are library books and children's magazines, but at times the reading materials may range from comic books to reference materials. The teacher helps the student select books and other materials of interest, checks the student's ability to independently read the materials, and conducts periodic, individual conferences with the student about the reading material. Typically, the teacher maintains records of the books read, date begun and completed, and some measure of the student's comprehension of the material. The comprehension measure may be an informal oral description or a written book report.

The major advantage of the individualized format to reading instruction is that each student reads on a topic of interest, at a rate, and on a level that is independent. Since within any classroom group there may be a range in mental age anywhere from 4 to 7 years, the major advantage of such a method is immediately apparent (Kirk, Kliebhan, & Lerner, 1978). There are other advantages. This approach can be initiated with any good books that are available and can inculcate the best in children's literature. The program can capitalize on the unique background and special interests of each student. Skills are taught as needed to the individual or in a small group. Therefore, the teacher can adjust the instruction to the student's optimal learning mode (see Figure 7).

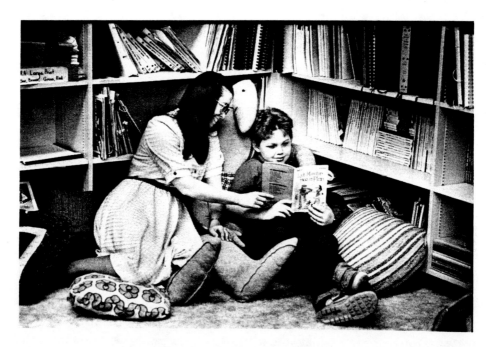

Figure 7. Individualized Format

The periodic individual conferences between teacher and student gives the student the feeling of importance and independence. During these conferences the teacher checks on comprehension and makes a note of any additional needs of instruction in basic skills. The student may read a portion of the material aloud to the teacher to give a diagnostic measure of the reading functioning level. Unless the group is very small, the limited conference times often allows insufficient time for adequate work with each student.

There are other disadvantages of the individualized approach for the visually impaired student. It probably makes more demands upon the teacher than any other reading format. The teacher must be ambitious, energetic, and knowledgeable of sequential reading skills. Considerable record keeping is required to document reading levels, to record books completed, and to monitor comprehension and accuracy. The teacher needs access to a large supply of books in braille and large print on many levels of difficulty and on a wide range of topics and must be a good organizer and manager of time.

In this format, there is no systematic procedure for the introduction and repetition of new vocabulary. There is no specific opportunity for developing readiness for new materials or for the group interaction so vital to the stimulation and growth of thinking skills. Some students have difficulty selecting materials appropriate to their reading levels.

The teacher of braille and large print readers may have difficulty providing a sufficient wealth of materials to match individual interests and reading levels. The teacher may find some children so passive that they have no initiative to get started or to propel themselves on a self-planned program. The individual format is probably not appropriate for such students. The individualized reading format is most useful with students who have mastered a sizable vocabulary and are independently motivated. The teacher may consider the use of the individual approach for some students for short, specific periods of time while other students in the group continue with another format. Another use of the individualized format is for a period, such as one grading period or one day per week. One teacher used the format in a project in which sixth graders became familiar with award winning books through braille, large print, cassettes, talking books, filmstrips, and videos.

The individualized format to reading instruction is based on sound principles and offers ideas that can be used to supplement any reading program. There are many ways in which a teacher can individualize much of the reading program, and the practical application of the principle of individualization can be incorporated within other reading formats.

Programmed Formats

Reading materials designed to teach reading skills in a programmed format are frequently published as cards or booklets. Programmed materials may provide some degree of individualization in reading instruction. Self-checking is usually a feature of programmed materials. Most include a record keeping system for teachers and some have placement tests. Teaching discrete and specific word identification or comprehension skills is a characteristic of most programmed materials. Testing for mastery and reteaching of each skill is built into some programmed materials. Although the content of the material is specifically prescribed, the learning is individualized in that students may progress through the program at different rates. These programmed materials may be the core of a reading program or may be used to supplement other programs.

Programmed materials, typically, are usable across several grade levels. They are sequenced according to difficulty, and that sequence is coded by some means such as color, letter, or symbol. Therefore, students can use them at many grade levels to meet their specific needs. Some of these materials are in book form, such as the Distar Instructional System, Specific Skill Reading Series, and the SRA Reading Laboratory Series and are available in braille from the American Printing House for the Blind.

Language-Experience Format

The language-experience format is a personalized approach to reading instruction. The content of the reading is based on some experience of the individual child or group, such as a field trip, a holiday party, or a game. The teacher and students discuss the experience and formulate a composite story recounting the sequence of events, the results of the experience, and their feelings concerning it. As the students relate the story, the teacher records it. This story then becomes the core of the reading lesson. Since the vocabulary and sentence construction are the students' own creation, many students can recognize their own sentences. After several of these experience stories, students begin to build a vocabulary of basic words which continues to grow from new experiences. Each student may have a collection of word cards for all words introduced to date, or a master list may be displayed or filed for teacher and student reference. The stories are usually recorded on classroom flip charts and retained for re-reading and review. They may be duplicated and made into individual booklets, one for each child. The latter plan, of course, would be preferable for the student using braille or large print.

The strongest advantage of this format is the integration of experience, oral language, written language, and reading. The words that are read carry the full and rich meaning of real personal experiences. Students build the concept that meaning is the core and purpose of reading.

Disadvantages of the language-experience format are that the student always knows the outcome, and there is no challenge to read to discover or think and predict the outcome of a story. Students may not be fully challenged with an exclusive language-experience format. The language-experience format does not control for the introduction or repetition of vocabulary. The introduction of phonemic elements and braille contractions is also not structured. Preparing the materials in the appropriate reading medium requires considerable teacher time and necessitates some delay between student diction and reading. The use of computer programs may assist the teacher in tallying the number of different words used and the number of times that word is used to help monitor the load of vocabulary. The computer may further personalize stories written by a group by printing each copy with the student's name. However, the advantage of providing reading material that relates to the visually impaired student's unique perception of experiences is an important advantage of the format.

An integrated language experience format for beginning reading may be especially advantageous to the visually impaired child who has little concept of the graphic symbols as representing meaning. Unlike the fully sighted preschool child, the visually impaired child has had little or no incidental exposure to words on signs, magazines, in picture books, and on television. The content in beginning reading materials may not be appropriate for the visually impaired student. The following example illustrates how reader content may be inappropriate.

> The first grade teacher was encouraging a group in outdoor activities. The teacher took the hand of Judy, an inactive, totally blind child, and suggested that they run together. Judy did not move and even resisted the slight pull that accompanied the second suggestion by the teacher that they run along the walk. In response to another persuasive attempt from the teacher, Judy replied, "I don't know what you mean." Judy had been delayed in beginning to walk; she had never run. She had never really interpreted the

sound of her little sister's running feet. Judy was not ready to read such sentence as, "Run, Ted, run!" She might have associated the verbal sound with the braille symbols. She might even have intonated the sentence with expression, mimicking the pattern of classmates. But Judy would have been engaging in a form of verbalism which has been found to be prevalent among blind individuals (Harley, 1963).

The language-experience format may be useful in the initial stages of reading to supplement or replace the print preprimers which are quite heavily dependent upon the picture context for meaning. The teacher can guide and supplement this approach to ensure a sufficient basic vocabulary for the students to enter the basal reading format at some specific level. In following such an approach, the teacher should plan experiences and activities that will provide the students with the opportunity for mastery of the words listed in the preprimers of that series or in some basic vocabulary list, such as those prepared by Johnson (1971), Dolch (1950), or Durr (1973).

Through the entire reading program, the teacher of visually impaired children must be especially alert to the need for meaningful experiences as a foundation for all reading. Fluent oral reading does not guarantee successful reading comprehension. The teacher should emphasize all of the comprehension skills, checking for responses in the student's own words to avoid parroting of words from the book.

SUMMARY

Each method and format of materials for the teaching of reading has its strong points; each has its pitfalls. Research does not validate the superiority of any one method, but tends more and more to indicate that the teacher is the important factor in the situation (Bond & Dykstra, 1967). There is no one "right" way to teach reading, but there are many right ways when selected and adapted to individual children. The teacher must constantly diagnose and prescribe, capitalizing on the child's optimal learning mode and strengthening other channels. The teacher of visually impaired children must have a thorough knowledge of the braille code characteristics which dictate unique approaches in the teaching of reading. These characteristics and adjustments are discussed in greater detail in Chapter 4.

CHAPTER 4

BUILDING WORD IDENTIFICATION SKILLS

THE PREVIOUS chapter presented an overview of various approaches to reading instruction and suggested some possible advantages and disadvantages of each approach for readers of braille or large print. The visually impaired student needs sequence and continuity in all aspects of communication development of which reading is a vital receptive channel.

The vision specialist may be guided, but not bound, by the organization ot the total school reading program. Emphasis on the individualization of learning through diagnostic-prescriptive teaching, behavior analysis, behavior objectives, and curriculum-based instruction benefit the visually impaired student as well as sighted classmates. The well-informed, creative teacher will analyze the reading process, diagnose student needs, and devise specific individualized teaching strategies which will maximize the student's learning opportunities.

The purpose of this chapter is to alert the teacher who will teach reading skills to readers of braille or large print regarding the unique characteristics of these media. The chapter does not purport to provide a comprehensive discussion of all word recognition and word attack skills. No attempt is made to duplicate the excellent presentations of the multiple aspects of reading which can be found in general textbooks on the subject. On the contrary, this chapter deals only with the manner in which these basic skills function in a unique way for the large print or braille reader. The authors strongly recommend that teachers of reading to visually impaired children have a secure foundation in the teaching of reading to normally seeing children since the skills used in teaching normally sighted children to read are the same skills that apply to visually impaired children. The first part of this chapter will focus on adaptations for print reading and the second part on braille reading.

PRINT FORMATS

When the vision teacher is providing instruction to low vision children who read large print, she will not have the challenge of adopting instruction through the braille code. The challenge for the teacher of visually impaired students is a continual process of assessment and modification with consideration of the student's visual efficiency and the student's interaction with the type size and style, contrast, page size, focal distance, optical aid, lighting, and time. Unlike the students who read braille and have the assurance that the braille characters in the textbook are the same size and shape as those they write or are written by the teacher, the low vision readers will be faced with an increasing variety of styles and sizes of print. The vision specialist's role is to monitor the student's progress and provide strategies by which the low vision student may read most quickly and accurately.

It may be helpful to the vision teacher to have an overview of he changes in format and type used by publishers of books for normally sighted children to better understand how these changes affect books that have been prepared for large print readers. The changes in format may include variances in type size, type styles, and spacing. Content may include punctuation, capitalization, vocabulary, and sentence length. These changes can be most difficult for the beginning reader. In general, the primary materials for the first through third grades are designed to help the student acquire a basic reading vocabulary that may be expanded through skills in phonics and structural analysis. Beyond the third grade the student is increasingly expected to use reading skills to acquire information in other subject areas.

Material in regular print at the first grade level is already enlarged for the normally sighted, beginning readers whose visual discrimination abilities are not fully developed. The majority of regular print publishers use larger type which is between 14 to 18 points in the preprimer books. When the type in these books is photo enlarged, the type size may be increased to 20-24 point type. By the beginning of the fourth grade, the type size in regular textbooks may be considerably reduced from the size that the student used in learning to read. Occasionally, at the end of the primary grades, a student may need to learn to use optical aids, such as closed curcuit television and listening equipment, such as talking books and cassette recorders.

Publishers of basal readers may use a variety of styles of type within a beginning book. The type style may change with each selection. For normally sighted students such changes may add variety, but for low vision students, words printed in a unique style may be unrecognizable. For a more complete discussion of changing type styles, see Chapter 6.

Spacing also affects readability. Preprimer books typically have been "slugged" in the printing process. This procedure leaves extra space between letters to make each letter more distinguishable from the letters on either side. For the low vision student who may need that extra space on each side of letters to determine the letter shape, the loss of the space in the primer or first level reader may make recognition of letters much more difficult.

PRINT CONTENT

Punctuation can be a confusing addition in large print or braille. For the normally seeing student, the admonition from the teacher to "don't pay any attention" to those marks may suffice, but for the reader of large print, the punctuation may be a very confusing addition to the letters in the adjacent words. Capitalization also alters the appearance of words. Print students may have success generalizing to capitalized words when the capitalized form is an enlargement of the lower case form, but they may have to learn to generalize capitalized words with significantly changed initial letter shapes, such as "go" and "Go."

Preprimers use very limited vocabularies of approximately 18-75 words. With such limited vocabularies, the length of sentences is abbreviated. A new sentence begins every line and each sentence ends a line. The concept of sentence "wrapping" may begin in the preprimers or may be delayed to the first reader. Even when the sentence is continued onto the next line for primer readers, it is broken at the end of a phrase, as in the example below:

> Bob went to the store
> to get a letter.

During beginning reading, the student is conditioned to think of the end of the line as the end of a sentence. With this expectation the student is predicting a "new sentence" word order rather than the continuation of a sentence on the next line.

The familiarity of the meaning of a word may be more important than the length or complexity of the word. To really "read" a word, the student must be able to say the word and to understand its meaning in the context. For example, the student who can correctly pronounce all the words in the following sentence: "Bill is fond of her." should be able to answer the question, "Did Bill like her?" If the meaning of "fond" is unfamiliar, the comprehension is lost.

The length of the sentence also affects the student's ability to read the sentence. The following sentence is relatively lengthy, but the order of words in the sentences is the same order as the sequence of events and is readable at a second grade level: "Helen said good-by to her dog every morning before the bus came." The sentence can be shorter with similar vocabulary but be more difficult to understand: "After petting the dog, Helen went to the bus." The basic idea of the two sentences is the same, but the first and longer sentence is easier to read.

The use of active or passive voice is important to the ease of understanding of a sentence. The following two sentences illustrate the influence of the active voice on the understanding: "The dog chased the cat." is in a active voice. "The cat was chased by the dog." uses the passive voice. The second sentence conveys the same meaning and adds only two words "was" and "by." Yet even though the two sentences are comparable by the most common measures of readability; namely, sentence length and the number of syllables in the word, they are definitely not comparable in terms of ease of comprehension. The active voice sentence is much more understandable.

The multiple meanings of words also contribute to readability. A student may be able to read the word "run" in isolation and in the context of a sentence where the meaning of the word is easily understood, as in the sentence, "Ruth can run to the house." However, recognition may be more difficult when other meanings of the word are used as in "home run," "water runs," or a "run" in a stocking.

At the end of the primary grades, students are expected to have basic decoding skills. Reading in applied areas such as science, social studies, and math increases greatly in sentence length and vocabulary complexity. For middle elementary grades, the readability difficulty of a science or social studies text may be one to two grade levels higher than the readability level of the basal reader from the same publisher. It is no wonder that teachers hear the complaint that Bobby can't read the science text. If the science text is written on a grade 5.4 reading level and Bobby is barely independent at a 4.1 reading level, then it is unlikely that he will be successful in understanding the content of the material even if he is able to laboriously decode the individual words.

The emphasis placed upon word identification in this chapter should not be misconstrued to imply that word recognition and reading are synonymous. Reading is the communication of ideas; it is a receptive aspect of language for the visually impaired reader of braille or large print as with fully sighted readers. Word recognition is the association of the printed form of the word with the sound. Reading comprehension involves the understanding of the meaning represented by the words and sentences. As a component of reading, word identification must preceed comprehension (Torgesen, 1986).

For the teacher initiating braille instruction, the teacher's own knowledge of the braille code and attitude toward braille reading have a significant impact upon the student's progress. The instructor must maintain a comfortable proficiency with reading and writing braille. The teacher may use the print copy of the reading materials by maintaining a mental picture of the format of the braille text and the unique structural elements of the code. In addition, the teacher may attempt a sufficient amount of finger reading to appreciate the difference between tactual and visual perception of the embossed characters. The teacher who has not mastered braille, who does not feel comfortable with the code, may unconsciously exert an adverse influence upon the learning process.

The major emphasis in this chapter is on tactual perception and braille reading since the majority of the unique teaching techniques are required for braille reading instruction. The teacher of the low vision student who is using print will have access to teaching strategies in the teacher's manual that parallels the student's book and in textbooks regarding reading instruction.

SIGHT WORD RECOGNITION

The development of word identification skills helps the visually impaired student to read more easily and efficiently. Word identification skills include sight word recognition, word analysis skills, and the use of context clues. These reading subskill areas are important for all readers including visually impaired readers. Teachers should be familiar with the general methods for teaching such skills to normally sighted children. The unique features of how to teach these skills to visually impaired children are largely due to the composition of the braille code.

The teacher who is working with both braille and print readers in the same group must be aware of the fact that recognition cues may be quite different for these two groups, and even confusing unless there is some clarification given. Words that are long in print may be short in braille due to the contracted forms of the code. For example, in braille the word "mother" appears to be no longer than "me"; "have" is shorter than "he," and "not" is shorter than "no." As noted in Figure 8, there are words such as "make" which have only the two single dots in the lowest position within the cell. These two single dots may be helpful recognition cues.

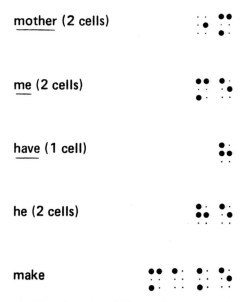

mother (2 cells)

me (2 cells)

have (1 cell)

he (2 cells)

make

Figure 8. Word length is different for print and braille.

Due to the contracted nature of the code, the braille reader needs a much greater store of instant words than does the reader of print. There are more than 150 braille words that contain insufficient elements to be recognized in any way other than by memory, aided by context. In texts designed for print readers, these special words may not receive sufficient repetition for mastery by the braille reader. Many of these words will be appearing at grade levels beyond those at which major attention is usually given to developing sight vocabulary. Therefore, the teacher must be aware of these words and devise activities that will insure their mastery.

The teacher should be familiar with the list of braille words which must be part of the reader's sight vocabulary. Some of these words are duplicates of those found in the Dolch list (see Figure 9 and appendix), but in some instances, such as the lower whole-word signs, the braille reader must master each word in two forms. For example, "was" is usually embossed in one cell as dots 3, 5, 6, but if it appears after a quotation mark it must be embossed in three cells using a symbol for each of its three letters.

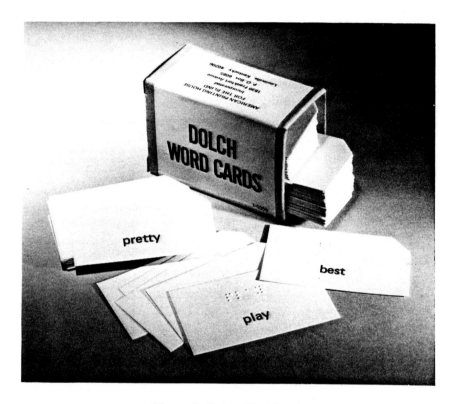

Figure 9. Dolch Word Cards

Familiar words may be grouped into five areas as follows:

1. Alphabet word signs: but, can, do, every, from, go, have, just, knowledge, like, more, not, people, quite, rather, so, that, us, very, will, it, you, as.
2. All initial-letter word signs (a) preceded by dot 5: day, ever, father, here, know, lord, mother, name, one, part, question, right, some, time, under, work, young, character, ought, there, through, where; (b) preceded by dots 4, 5: upon, word, these, those whose; and (c) preceded by dots 4, 5, 6: cannot, had, many, spirit, world, their.
3. One-cell whole-word signs: and, for, of, the, with, child, shall, this, which, still, out.

4. Lower whole-word signs: enough, were, his, in, into, by, was, to. These words must also be mastered in full spelling because, according to the rules of the code, they appear in both forms.
5. Short-form words: about, above, according, across, after, afternoon, afterward, again, against, almost, already, also, altogether, although, always, because, before, behind, below, beneath, beside, between, beyond, blind, braille, children, conceive, conceiving, could, deceive, deceiving, declare, declaring, either, first, friend, good, great, herself, him, himself, immediate, its, itself, letter, little, much, must, myself, necessary, neither, o'clock, oneself, ourselves, paid, perceive, perceiving, perhaps, quick, receive, receiving, rejoice, rejoicing, said, should, such, themselves, thyself, today, together, tomorrow, tonight, would, your, yourself, yourselves.

Appendix B, Behavioral Objectives of the Braille Code, provides guidelines for selecting teaching objectives for reading and writing braille. Mastery of the code is organized in grade levels first through sixth.

WORD ANALYSIS SKILLS

The purpose of this section is to identify where instruction in word analysis differs for the visually impaired braille reader. Additional suggestions for adaptive techniques for readers of braille and large print are discussed in Chapters 7 and 12.

Phonics

In addition to the sight-words which are needed in reading, visually impaired students need word analysis skills in identifying unfamiliar words that may become sight words with practice. Reading specialists may not agree on the exact sequence of steps, including the phonic rules, in learning to analyze words. however, the condensed list included here is a sequence of steps that has proven to be effective in teaching reading to normally sighted and visually impaired children (Kirk, Kliebhan, & Lerner, 1978, & Truan, 1978).

Steps in Learning to Analyze Words

1. Sounds of single consonants: s, b, t
2. Sounds of consonant blends: bl, br, cl, dr, sm, str

3. Sounds of consonant diagraphs: ch, sh, th, wh
4. Short sounds of vowels: a, e, i, o, u
5. Final "e" rule for long vowel sounds: cake, ripe
6. Double vowels: ai, ay, ee, ea, oa
7. Variant vowels: oi, oy, ou, ow, eu, ew, oo, o͞o
8. Sounds of vowels with "r:" ar, or, er, ir, ur
9. Short "c" and "g" before e, i, and y
10. Recognize common prefixes and suffixes
11. Try as many syllables as vowel sounds
12. Divide syllables between two consonants or in front of one consonant.
13. Syllable ends in vowel, try long vowel; syllable ends in consonant, try short vowel.

The first nine steps in the word analysis list are typically described as phonics in the literature. The last four steps are usually identified as structural analysis and syllabication. Appendix B, Word Identification Skills by Grade Level K-6, contains an expanded sequence of these word analysis skills to assist the teacher in planning instruction.

The number of phonic rules that should be taught is limited. Spache (1963), on the basis of extensive research, lists the rules that pass the criterion of 75% utility and dependability. These rules apply regardless of the reading medium. However, many of the phonic rules concerning vowel control rely on cues that follow rather than precede the vowel. Since fingers traverse the reading line more slowly than do the eyes, these cues are not as spontaneously applicable for the braille reader as for the print reader.

Phonemic cues are important in identification of unfamiliar words. These cues consist not only of the letter-sound associations, but also the recognition of common phonemic elements or groups that occur frequently within the words of our language. These orthographic cues function in coordination with the semantic and syntactic signals, confirming or rejecting the reader's best guess at a word not instantly recognized.

Research seems to indicate that rapid phonetic synthesis is a skill essential to the braille reading process. As a result of a series of studies, Nolan and Kederis (1969) concluded that braille word identification is accomplished by just such a process over a temporal-spatial span, as noted in Chapter 3.

One of the learner's earliest steps in the application of phonics to word identification is the discovery of sound-symbol relationships for initial consonants. Children discover that words in a given group which sound the same at the beginning also look the same at the beginning. Several factors make this discovery a little more difficlt for the braille reader than for one who reads print. The formation of braille letters within the 6-dot cell results in some open, broken characters. Thus, dots within adjacent letters appear tactually to have more of an entity than do the dots within the letter. Also, characteristic of the code are the prefixed dots which have no sound of their own, but which tend to obscure the tactual perception of the accompanying letter.

Consider the letter "m" which is usually one of the first consonants introduced. Note the openness of the configuration. The dots 1 and 4 frequently appear more closely related to the letter which follows than they do to the dot 3 at the bottom of the cell. The word "mother" may be used by some authors as a key word in this discovery of sound-symbol relationship. Yet in braille "Mother" has two prefixed dots which confuse the configuration of "m" as the initial symbol. As may be seen in Figure 10, the annexation of the symbol for the word "to" in such common phrases as "to me" and "to mother" adds the possibility of further confusion because the symbol for "to" is written next to "me" or "mother" without an intervening space.

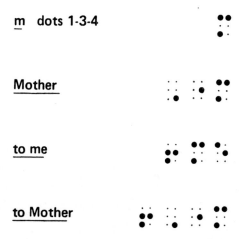

Figure 10. Variable configurations with the letter "m."

During the process of teaching initial sounds, the teacher will find it advantageous to provide for the braille reader sufficient contacts with the letter in isolation to insure adequate familiarity with its configuration. Of course, the teacher who is dealing with only braille readers may be selective and utilize first those letters which have fewer confusing elements, reserving the more complex situations until the child has more skill. Although not all authorities agree, many teachers find the teaching of dot numbers for the configuration to be beneficial in establishing clear concepts and in discouraging the tendency to reversals of perceptual images. The inclusion of dot numbers is helpful if reading and writing instruction are initiated together.

Most alphabet word signs can be utilized in teaching initial consonant sounds. However, there are some pitfalls to be avoided. The letter "f" stands for "from," which begins with the "fr" blend and not the pure "f" sound. Since no common words begin with the letters "x" or "z," these letters have been assigned the meanings of "it" and "as" and, therefore, have no initial sound-symbol relationship. The letter "t" is the worst confuser among the alphabet word signs because it represents "that," which has the initial letter but not the "t" sound. Students sometimes have difficulty learning this word because of this phonic violation.

Consonant substitution does not always function alike for braille and print readers. For example, specialists writing materials for print readers can assume that, after the reader knows "work," the process of consonant substitution will aid him in recognizing "word," and the inclusion of one more familiar sound component will give "world." For the braille reader the only phonetic elements in any of these words is the "w." Each word must be memorized as a part of the instant vocabulary.

Some special considerations may be necessary in teaching rhyming words, or word families. For example, "can," "not," "that," "will," and "it" are words frequently included in building word families. Of course, in each cited case, the graphic representation of the word family does not exist in the braille form. If any of these words are to be used as the basis for discovering word families, the child must be taught the full spelling. A better approach might be to use other words as the basis for discovering the word family. Then, show the child the alphabetic word sign that belongs within that family. The teacher may challenge a sharp student to discover how to spell the contracted word. For example, in the words "an," "man," and "ran," the child is led to discover the graphics and sound of the "an" family. Then add to the list "can," which in braille is represented by "c." After the child pronounces all the words in the list, the spelling of "can" may be discovered.

Although the final-letter signs of the braille code all represent very convenient common phonograms, once they are mastered, there can be some confusion during the learning process. Each of these signs contains the consonant representing the final letter sound instead of the initial sound. Students who have become fairly automatic in their application of initial consonant sounds tend to respond to the consonant within the sign as though it were initiating the phonogram. Thus, they have to overcome the tendency to identify dots 5-6, "l" as "less" instead of "ful." They name dots 4-6, "n," as "ness" instead of "sion," and dots 5-6, "s," as "sion" instead of "ness." Sufficient drill must be planned to insure correct, rapid identification of the final-letter signs.

These phonetic idiosyncracies of the braille code in no way negate the value of phonics as a word identification skill for the finger reader. The teacher must maintain competence with braille in order to guide the student in the most effective use of phonics as related to the embossed code.

The teacher may also capitalize on a number of elements of the code that facilitate the application of phonic skills. Some of the common consonant blends and diagraphs are represented by single characters in braille. These include "ch," "sh," "th," "st," "gh," and "wh." Note also common vowel diphthongs and diagraphs such as "ea," "ou," "ow," and the "r"-controlled units "ar" and "er." Other braille contractions represent many useful phonograms. It is essential that the language arts program provide adequate instructional activities to insure the instant recognition of braille characters and their component sounds.

Structured Analysis

In many ways structural analysis functions as a word attack skill for the braille reader just as it does for the reader of print. Using structural analysis, the reader breaks the word into meaningful parts. Instruction of structural analysis progresses from recognition of words that have been expanded with inflectional endings, combined in compound words, combined with prefixes, suffixes, to other root words within multiple syllable words.

Some special considerations are necessary for the beginning reader who is working with sighted peers or with materials that are exact transcriptions from print texts. Frequently, authors of early reading series do not consider a root word with an inflectional ending as a new word. If a child knows "like," then "likes" does not have to be treated as a new word with the designated amount of repetition assigned to new words. For the braille reader, such variants frequently do appear to be entirely new. In the foregoing example in Figure 11, "like" appears as "l," whereas "likes" would be in full spelling. For the braille reader, the word identification process may at times mean learning two instant words instead of recognizing a known root word and an inflectional ending, illustrated in Figure 11.

BRAILLE CONTRACTIONS
&
STRUCTURAL ANALYSIS

Unhelpful in Structural Analysis

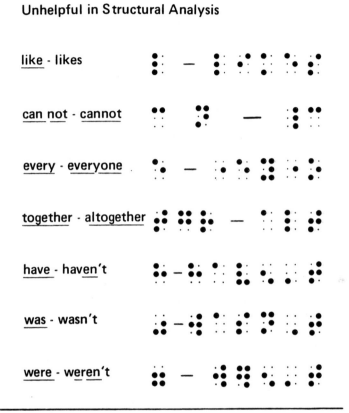

Helpful in Structural Analysis

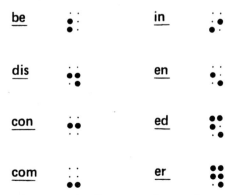

Figure 11. Braille contractions and structural analysis.

The forms of some braille words are altered substantially when they become parts of compound words. For example, "cannot" does not appear to be the combination of "can" and "not," but is an entirely new form that must be mastered as a sight word. The word "every" must be written as dot 5, "e" and "y." "Child" is "ch" when alone but is spelled out as part of a compound word. Every one of the alphabet word signs must change in form to be combined with another word. "Tgr," which is read as "together," is no help in identifying "altogether," which is "alt" in braille. The reader must recognize a change in form in some allographs, such as "haven't," "wasn't," and "weren't," since "have," "was," and "were" have special whole-word signs when written alone.

Syllabication may not be as effective for the finger reader as for the print reader. Braille contractions are used freely to cross all syllable divisions except those occurring between prefixes or suffixes and root words, between parts of compound words, and in some exceptional words such as "airedale," in which the sign would confuse pronunciation. Thus, syllable divisions are frequently obscured. However, Spache (1976) points out that strict adherence to syllabication is not essential for word identification. The reader can look for perceptual units or pronounceable parts within unknown words. Once an individual has mastered the numerous braille contractions, then the contractions usually serve adequately as perceptual units or pronounceable parts of words. Some confusers are words such as "sofa" and "zero," in which the "o" of "of" and the "e" in "er" each have the long vowel sound because it ends a c-v, or open syllable. The word "partial" is another example of a situation in which the reader must respond instantly not only to the tactual unit but also to its component letters to apply accurate syllabication and achieve correct pronunciation.

The reader visually determines the number of syllables or pronounceable parts within a word by the number of vowel sounds. A few of the short form words, such a "herf" (herself) and "alt" (altogether) contain one vowel. The reader may perceive them as one-syllable words and pronounce them as such. Such words need to be taught as part of the sight vocabulary. For the braille reader, the mastery of instant vocabulary may be an essential part of the language arts program over a greater span of years than is necessary for the print reader.

Situations in which the orthography of the braille code alters the structure of words need present no great difficulty for the braille reader when the teacher is competent with the code and helps the student to utilize the appropriate word identification skills. The teacher should be thoroughly familiar with braille to avoid inappropriate instruction. For example, a teacher was using the print copy of the text in a class of print and braille readers when a braille reader faltered on the word "immediate." The teacher directed: "It sounds exactly like it is spelled. Divide it up and sound it out." Of course, such a suggestion was confusing to the child who perceived only "imm." The teacher finally had another child, who read print, read the word. A more effective procedure would have been to tell the child that the word was one of the shortforms in braille and to help the student use the semantic and syntactic context clues along with the beginning sound in order to predict what the word might be.

Some characteristics of the braille code may aid the reader in structural analysis. Contractions may serve as perceptual units and pronounceable parts of words. Some of the signs represent meaningful prefixes and suffixes. Note the signs for "be," "con," "com," "dis," and "in," as illustrated in Figure 11. The final-letter signs represent common suffixes. Inflected word endings are "ed," "ing," and "er." These signs, which represent prefixes, suffixes, and inflected endings, have a high utility. Some of the prefixes and most of the suffixes appear infrequently in books prior to the third grade. Therefore, this aspect of structural analysis is an important part of the language arts program in third and fourth grades.

Context Clues

Efficient readers develop the ability to make optimum use of semantic and syntactic context clues for word identification. These skills relate most directly to the purpose of the reading process. As visually impaired readers respond to context clues, they also develop comprehension skills. Effective application of context clues is an indicator that the individual is reading for meaning.

The mature print reader relies much more upon context clues than upon detailed word analysis (Goodman, 1973). This shift in major attention from detailed word analysis to greater reliance upon context clues usually occurs by the time the student reaches the upper elementary level. The same shift to reliance on context clues appears true for visually impaired readers of large print and braille.

Both the semantic and syntactic clue systems of oral language offer clues about unfamiliar words. Syntactic clues lie within our language structure. English sentences are ordered in such a way that we expect certain types of words to occur in certain positions. Semantic clues lie within the associated meanings of words, phrases, clauses, and sentences. To illustrate, consider the following incomplete sentence: The big dog _____ . If asked to complete this sentence, a child would probably name an active verb because in English grammar the verb falls in that position. This expectancy is the syntactic clue. The student would probably select a word such as barked, growled, or jumped because these words are associated with the concept of dog. This association of meaning is the semantic clue. The reader responds to these same syntactic and semantic clues when an unfamiliar word is encountered.

Identification of the graphic symbols or letters is the first step in learning to read. Misidentification of the letters and/or their order almost precludes entry into steps two and three in reading. After identifying the letters, the second step in reading is to translate the letters into sound or spoken language. Subvocalization (reading with a whisper or lip movement) during reading is a common characteristic of students through the primary grades. The third step of reading occurs when the spoken sound is translated into concept or meaning. Very proficient, older readers may eventually skip step two, which means printed symbols would be directly translated into ideas. This uncommon proficiency may be evidenced by the large number of well-educated readers whose reading speeds never exceed that of rapid speech. The greatest difficulty for the beginning reader of braille or large print is that preschool experiences may not have prepared them to use context to identify words.

The child must discover the concept that an object represented by letters is not the same regardless of position of the letters in the sentence. Previous experience has not prepared the child for this multiplicity of meaning of words. The child knows that a shoe is a shoe regardless of its position or setting. It may be on the foot, in the mother's hand, in the back of the closet, on the floor of the car, in the toy box, or half-eaten by the family pet. Whether new or damaged, backward or forward, upside down, horizontal, or bent, the child recognizes the shoe. The identity of letters is not so constant. The letter name and sound may change in print or braille by the relative position with other letters and words and the direction in which it is turned.

Entering the first grade, the visually impaired child has had relatively little experience with linear objects. The world has largely been a three-dimensional world of objects and people. The child has had relatively little experience with two-dimensional linear objects of which letters and numbers are made. Even with two-dimensional objects, such as circles, squares, and triangles, the child has been taught to recognize them regardless of their placement.

As children enter the first step in learning to read, they encounter a learning task which they could not logically anticipate from previous learning. A configuration positioned in any pattern of lines or dots that is different may become a different letter entirely. For example, the shape "d" representing the sound /d/ may be perceived by the low vision reader as letters "p," "b," and "q." Similarly, reversing the sequence of letters can make a new word, such as in "saw" and "was." Even for the young print reader with no perceptual damages, this "reversal" problem is frequently seen in the early stages of learning to read. By the middle of the first grade, normally sighted children without perceptual damage rarely make incorrect orientations in reading and/or writing. (Kirk, Kliebhan, & Lerner, 1978).

The braille reader must respond to unique context clues that arise from the internal structure of the code itself. These clues deal primarily with the spatial variables. For example, the right-angle shape composed of two dots in a left vertical position and one dot to the right bottom of these two can be composed of either dots 1-2-5 or of dots 2-3-6. The reader will not know which set of dots has been used unless the reader can orient that shape in relation to other braille characters. If the shape contains dots 2-3-6, the student must continue to use the spatial context to make further decisions. If this shape precedes another character without any intervening space, it is an opening quotation mark. If a space occurs on each side of the uncapitalized symbol, it is the word "his." If it follows another character with no intervening space, it is a question mark as illustrated in Figure 12.

Suppose the shape under consideration is composed of dots 1-2-5. If this shape is preceded and followed by a space, it is the word "have." If it is immediately adjacent to any letter or contraction, it is interpreted as the letter "h." Should the reader be dealing with mathematics, the same symbol becomes the numeral "8." Within the context of music, it becomes the note "G."

The braille reader meets numerous situations in which the interpretation of the symbol depends upon the discernment of the spatial context as well as upon the content area involved. The student needs to develop maximum use of as many fingers as possible in order to cover a sufficient span to provide spatial information. The smooth, left-to-right hand movement also aids in this correct interpretation.

SIMILAR BRAILLE CONFIGURATIONS

2-3-6		opening quotation mark
⠒		his
		question mark
		numeral 8 (Nemeth Code)

1-2-5		letter h
⠓		have
		numeral 8 (literary numbers)
		note G (music notation)

Figure 12. Similar braille configuration.

The use of context is a major source of information in interpreting reversible letters and words for the print or braille reader. However, use of context is most essential to the braille reader. Context clues play a major role from the earliest stages of reading, when the child is building a sight vocabulary. The teacher may use a language-experience story which relies on a recent meaningful experience to supply a strong semantic context. Since the story is written in the child's own language pattern, the syntactic context is provided. These two sets of clues are a strong support of word identification.

Adequate application of semantic and syntactic context clues is one of the most effective aids to word identification in approaching an unknown or unfamiliar word. The mind responding to these clues predicts a word that will be acceptable both in meaning and in grammatical form. Thus, these clues create an expectancy or mind set for the unknown word which can then be verified by word analysis.

On the preprimer and primer levels of print reading series, the pictures supply most of the plot. The print reader receives semantic clues for the picture. In fact, some print readers depend so heavily upon the picture clues that, if the pictures are covered, they have difficulty reading the book. The braille reader is at a disadvantage because the picture clues are not present.

The teacher may collect objects that will appear within the first few books so that the children can handle them and become familiar with their appearance and their functions. Three-dimensional scenes from within the stories can be constructed and examined tactually by the children. The skillful teacher can guide the group into constructing the plot that will appear in the story. Some stories lend themselves to dramatization as a means of familiarizing students with the basic plot. The students may be the actors or use puppets or dolls. Another possibility is for the teacher to tell the story in a dramatic way, letting the students read the lines from the book at the appropriate spots. A few braille readers may be able to see pictures or picture parts in the regular print book.

Describing the pictures to braille readers may provide little meaningful context. Many visually impaired children have limited backgrounds of experience and are more oriented to themselves. They may not be able to project themselves into a verbalized setting. The constant reference to the pictures reminds the braille students that sighted peers have a source of informaion not available to them. One first grader was able to verbalize the feeling: "This makes me so mad! Don't they know we want to find out things for ourselves!"

A good plan to build word anticipation and use of context is through a discussion of the story title and any introductory paragraph that may provide an understanding of the story setting. Students can list words that they think might be found in such a passage. This word expectancy growing out of context clues aids the students in recognizing vocabulary in reading. The syntax of the book may be far more complex than the normal language pattern of the students. Guided class study time may be necessary in order to help students learn to interpret the language structure of the textbook.

The "cloze technique" can be used either to increase the use of context clues or as an instrument to assess skills in utilizing context clues. Every tenth noun or verb is usually omitted from a short story. Students read the story and supply acceptable words for the blanks. The task may be increased by omitting every fifth noun or verb, and then by omitting every fifth or tenth word regardless of the type of word. Unrelated sentences may be used instead of a continuous story. Through selection of the type of omission within the activity, practice can be given in the application of any type of context clue whether semantic or syntactic. Spache (1976) claims that, if the material is on the student's reading level, the student should select the exact word of the original reading passage for at least two out of every five cloze omissions.

Another factor may affect the manner in which context clues function for the braille reader. The brain tends to process meaning more rapidly than the fingers perceive the tactual stimuli. Therefore, the brain seeks clozure before the fingers reach the tactual clues. The brain may supply a word that is semantically and syntactically satisfactory, but as the fingers reach the graphic symbols the prediction proves to be inaccurate, and the mental pattern must be revised. Ashcroft (1960) called attention to the fact that braille readers must suspend judgment before clozure to a greater degree than do print readers in order to reduce errors.

DICTIONARY

In identifying unfamiliar words, the visually impaired reader can utilize the dictionary as a source of information. Large print dictionaries are oversized but frequently are contained in one volume. A one volume version may have somewhat abbreviated entry information to maintain the total number of words. The dictionary may serve as a good reference for the braille reader although it may not be as conveniently available as in the print copy. A vest pocket dictionary in print is quite compact, but a braille edition consists of seven volumes and requires almost two feet of shelving. Not only does this bulk limit the number of copies that may be available, it also means that the dictionary is cumbersome to use. The availability of dictionaries through audible cassette tape, paperless braille cassette, and computer programs, which are accessible through the speech snynthesizer, should make the dictionary more accessible in terms of space and time.

The teacher will need to carefully plan activities to develop the skills necessary for efficient use of the braille dictionary. In lieu of the picture dictionaries commercially available for early readers of print, object dictionaries may be devised for the braille reader. Any classroom that has a set of Tactual Aids to Reading (Caton, 1974) produced by the American Printing House for the Blind has an excellent readiness tool. The objects in this collection are packaged alphabetically in a set of drawers. Each drawer contains objects representing two or three initial letter sounds. The drawers can be labeled with the appropriate braille letters. Children may help locate and replace objects that are used in various activities. They may learn that an object such as the wheel belongs in a drawer near the bottom of the case, whereas an apple will be placed in the first drawer. This early association of the letters in their relative position within the alphabet is good preparation for the later use of the many volumes of the braille dictionary.

Students can become acquainted with the elements of a dictionary through the creation of simple classroom card files. These files might contain new vocabulary words from field trips, social studies, and science. Each card could contain a word with its definition. Cards are filed alphabetically upside down, and from the back to the front of the box. This arrangement makes it possible for the braille reader to reach into the box, locate the desired card, and read it without removing it from the box.

Classroom or individual card file dictionaries increase in their complexity as the student develops skills. Various grammatical forms may be included, each with its correct designation. Phonetic spelling can be introduced.

Many reading activities, such as alphabetization, syllabication, and selection of appropriate meanings will be similar for all readers whether using print or braille. However for the braille reader activities that involve the location of a letter within its relative segment of the alphabet are especially valuable. A student must know the approximate location of a word to avoid wasting much valuable time and becoming very frustrated attempting to use the many volumes of the braille dictionary. The student also needs experience in utilizing the guide words on the volume cover as an aid to rapid location of a word.

During the braille reader's initiation into the use of a diacritical mark, consistency in both terminology and graphics is needed. Textbooks in English, reading, and spelling usually include instruction and practice in dictionary skills. A great amount of variation in the terms used to identify sound elements and in the manner of marking such sounds can be found frequently among these texts. During the initial stages of instruction for the braille reader, texts that agree in their diacritical markings should be employed. Eventually the student will find it necessary to interpret a variety of diacritical symbols as well as differing definitions of sound units. Since the braille diacritics involve symbols exactly like those used for letters and contractions in the literary code, the student should not initially be required to meet the proliferation of symbols introduced by various lexicographers. Each braille text will contain a key to pronunciation to aid the reader in interpretation of the markings employed within that text.

DEVELOPING GOOD MECHANICS

Unlike the eyes of a normal seeing child, the fingers of a blind child have not been constantly stimulated throughout the preschool years. The environment challenges and motivates the eyes; fingers must seek out the environment. Some visually impaired children have very poor musculature resulting from additional handicaps or merely from years of inertia. Developing muscle tone in both large and small muscles may precede work on the development of the fine muscular attention and coordination essential for the tactual perception of braille.

Although for convenient reference the mechanics of touch reading are discussed in detail at this point, they should not be taught in a detailed and formalized manner. The teacher will demonstrate, describe, and suggest techniques as applicable but will maintain the focus of attention on reading for meaning. Praise for the child who is using good techniques, such as the child in Figure 13, may motivate others to imitate.

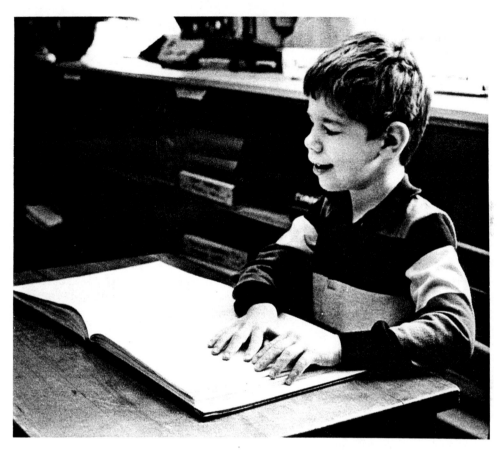

Figure 13. Developing good mechanics for braille reading.

Various researchers (Burklen, 1932; Maxfield, 1928; & Eatman, 1942) cite characteristics of efficient braille readers. However, there is evidence of a variety of techniques among very effective readers. The results of a survey by Lowenfeld, Abel, and Hatlen (1969) showed that even though students had been taught specific techniques during their primary years, by the time they reached eighth grade they have assumed book and hand positions and hand functioning most comfortable to each of them. Although the use of both hands independently is the recommended reading style for most braille readers, there is some research to indicate that no relationship exists between particular style and frequency of errors (Davidson, Wiles-Kettermann, Haber, & Appelle,

1980). However the teacher should be aware of pertinent information concerning tactual reading and should encourage the student to establish certain proven techniques until good reading habits are well established.

The hand position should make the most efficient use of the pads of the fingers on the reading surface since the maximum sensitivity is in the pads. The fingers curved comfortably allow the pads to focus major attention on the upper part of the cell, where the majority of dots appear, but also to span the entire 3-dot depth of the cell. Maxfield (1928) suggested an approximate 30 degree angle with the page. The angle, however, will differ with the size of the hand. For the child's initial encounter with lines of braille, the teacher may suggest and demonstrate to the child to bring both hands together with the thumbs gently touching and with the upper joints of the index fingers in light contact with each other. Fingers may slide quickly and easily from left to right. Practice with only one line of braille is helpful while the child is establishing this position. The tips of all eight fingers, or at least the first three on each hand, should rest lightly on the reading line. If the child's little fingers are unusually short, attempts to maintain all eight fingers on the reading line may result in forcing the other fingers onto the fingertips and not allow the spanning of the entire depth of the cell. A straight wrist position is preferable.

Braille is perceived through the pressure points within the surface of the finger pads. A light and even pressure is conducive to good perception. A heavier pressure spreads the perception points and blurs the image. The normal tendency to increase the pressure when perception is difficult only compounds the problem. Burklen (1932) found that touch movements of good readers proceeds in a straight running line with slight and uniform pressure on the fingers. He found the touch movements of poorer readers occurred in serrated or twisting movements with stronger and more unsteady pressure on the fingers. Holland (1934) noted that fast readers tend to use less pressure than slow readers, but that pressure varied with less pressure in the beginning than at the end of a line or, especially in poor readers, at the end of a paragraph.

In an experiment by Kusajima (1974), the relationship between up and down movements and pressure was studied. He found that expert readers who make few up-and-down or flutter movements with their fingers also moved their fingers with almost uniform pressure over all the cells of the braille line. The same proficient readers demonstrated uneven pressure with nonsense words, just as poor readers had uneven pressure on all material. The high correlation between pressure and up-and-down or flutter movements was evidenced by the markings on a pressure recording drum. Some slight increases in pressure were noted by better readers at some braille cells but the best readers read whole lines with uniform low pressures. The teacher may demonstrate "light pressure" by placing the hands in the reading position and sliding them lightly along the child's arm. The teacher may ask the child to do the same. Perspiring or whitening fingers usually indicates too much pressure. If the teacher suspects too much tension or pressure, the teacher may gently place a hand under the child's wrist and lift slightly.

As many fingers as possible should be utilized in the reading process. Lowenfeld, Abel, and Hatlen (1969) found that most students utilize the index finger or the index and middle fingers on one or both hands as the primary reading fingers. Other fingers serve to maintain orientation on the braille line, to check punctuation, and to move between lines.

An informal activity for the beginning reader who is using only the index fingers in contact with the page begins with the preparation of a paper in which eight pipestem cleaner sections of varying lengths are placed vertically so that each of the child's eight fingers touches one section. The child is asked to move the hands down the page touching the fuzzy cleaners and to tell when one finger reaches the end of a section. Commercially available materials that encourage the use of all fingers have been developed by Mangold (1978) called the *Mangold Developmental Program of Tactile Perception and Braille Letter Recognition* and by Kurzhals & Caton (1974) called the *Tactual Road to Reading*.

Eatman (1942) found that the coordinated use of both hands was characteristic of the majority of the best readers. While the right hand was completing one line the left hand moved to the beginning of the next line to continue the reading. The two hands then met at some point approaching the middle of the new line, and once again separated to perform their separate but coordinated functions. Eatman found that on the average 7% of the total reading time was consumed in return sweeps to new reading lines. Therefore, any technique that will facilitate this transition would greatly improve reading speed.

Fertsch (1946), in using filmed records to study 63 subjects, noted that good readers were those whose hands functioned independently of each other. Two variations in making return sweeps were noted. The good readers moved their hands to the beginning of the new line independently of each other and without retracing a line of braille. The poor readers retraced a line of braille with one or both of their hands to find the beginning of the next line. Fertsch concluded that it would be desirable to teach pupils to move directly to the beginning of a new line without tracing a line of braille.

Lowenfeld, Abel, and Hatlen (1969) noted that eighth graders who read ahead on the next line with the left hand while the right hand finished the preceding line tended to be the more efficient readers. They concluded that readers who use both hands should be encouraged to use this procedure. Crandell and Wallace (1974) suggested innovative hand movements such as a pattern starting with the hands at the center of the line. Although they found higher speeds of braille reading with 6 days of rapid reading training with adults, there were so many variables that the effect of the hand movement instruction could not be measured. Olson (1977), after completing a doctoral dissertation on rapid reading training with adults, suggested that the teacher take the student's hand and demonstrate how the two hands can be used together or independently over a page. Another suggestion was that students can be taught to continue reading with one hand while the other hand turns a page to increase reading speed.

Eatman (1942) measured the ability of the right hand and the left hand, each functioning alone. She then measured the ability of both hands functioning together. The readers whose scores with the independent right hand and the independent left hand were almost equal tended to be among the most efficient readers when the two hands functioned together. The teacher can devise activities to develop the effectiveness of each hand, such as a worksheet containing two columns of words or symbols. The reader will move simultaneously down the left column with the left hand and the right column with the right hand, stating whether the items in each pair are the same or different. Another activity would be to compile a list of words on the left, and either their synonyms or antonyms in mixed order in a list on the right. The student would read the word with the left hand and keep a finger on that word while with the right hand scan the other list for the synonym or antonym as directed. For variety, the stimulus list might be on the right, necessitating the scanning with the left hand. The teacher may suggest that a student complete the reading of the final line on a page with one hand while beginning the line at the top of the next page with the other hand.

Quick, smooth left-to-right hand movements are characteristic of efficient braille readers. For the sighted reader, visual perception occurs as the eye pauses, but for the braille reader tactual perception is achieved through movement across the symbols.

Various activities can motivate the quick scanning of the braille line. Reading a personal news item, an experience story, a favorite nursery rhyme or poem, as the teacher reads aloud, encourages fingers to glide smoothly. On the primary reading level the teacher may read a sentence or short paragraph aloud while the children follow in their books. The teacher will stop before some significant word, such as a noun, verb, or adjective to see if the children can first supply the next word. The children will attempt to keep pace with the teacher's voice so that they may read the designated word. The child may be stimulated to move fingers quickly and join classmates in reading a short passage silently to find a word or phrase to answer a specific question.

When reading a word or phrase card or when moving to a new reading line, the student should be discouraged from retracing the braille line from right to left. The retracing of the stimulus pattern in reverse may increase reversal problems. When reading words on a card, the student may lift the fingers to return to the beginning. When moving to a new braille line the student may move in the space just under the line completed.

Several methods have been successfully used to increase reading speed of braille readers. These methods include:

1. Practicing character recognition (Henderson, 1967; Umsted, 1970).
2. Using programmed machine pacing device (Flanigan & Joslin, 1969).
3. Giving feedback on reading speed (Crandell & Wallace, 1974; Olson, Harlow, & Williams, 1975; Truan, 1978).
4. Practicing tracking and return sweeps (Olson, Harlow, & Williams, 1975; Mangold, 1978; Wormsly, 1981).

All of these methods have been researched with braille readers and they have proven to be successful. An important element which probably involves all events is "motivation." If the teacher really convinces the children that her method will work in increasing reading speed, it should be of valuable assistance in improving braille reading speed of the students.

The teacher is responsible for providing a good reading environment that will motivate and encourage good habits. This includes a relaxed and positive learning atmosphere in which each child feels accepted. Although it is imperative that the teacher exercise good classroom management and control; there should be no feeling of fear or tension. Any such feeling inhibits the relaxed smooth functioning of the reading fingers.

Good room ventilation is important; fresh air in a well-ventilated room stimulates both physical and mental alertness. Neither cold hands nor hot, perspiring hands function efficiently. Washing in warm or cold water immediately prior to the reading period may help braille reading efficiency.

The furniture in the room affects the braille reader's reading posture. The reading surface should be of sufficient size to support the entire book and should be no higher than the elbow level of the reader. A reading surface above elbow level causes either a hunching of shoulders or a spreading of elbows that places the reader's hands into a awkward reading position.

Interest in reading encourages good habits. The teacher's own enthusiasm for reading is contagious. Classroom reading centers with textured, easy to read books on a variety of subjects create reading interests. Easy to read books encourage rapid, smooth hand movements. All braille should be of good quality because errors in braille and rubbed-out dots encourage scrubbing motions of the fingers.

A high degree of sensitivity in the fingers is not essential to good braille reading. In fact, many avid readers have slightly calloused fingers. Eatman (1942) suggests that unless an individual possesses some extreme disability in touch he can become an effective reader. Highly motivated students who for some reason did not have the use of their hands have been known to learn to read using the tongue or the toes. Readers display individual perferences for the height of the braille dots. Some students prefer dots that are relatively low and rounded. They will, if possible, avoid the use of a new braille book, stating that the high dots irritate their fingers.

SUMMARY

This chapter has dealt with some of the unique methods and instructional strategies available to teachers of students reading large print or braille. The effects of format and content changes required to provide material in large print preceded a description of suggested instructional techniques to develop whole-word identification, word analysis skills, context clues, and use of the dictionary. Although the chapter treated each reading skill separately, these skills cannot be separated in the reading process. They function simultaneously, interacting to check, support, confirm, or correct.

Semantic and syntactic context cues are essential. They function to a high degree during the initial steps in reading, as the child relies upon oral language cues to give meaning to new graphic forms of communication. The mature reader also depends highly upon these cues. Attention focuses on phonic and structural word analysis (orthographic cues) during the primary years. The mature reader, faced with very difficult material reverts back to a reliance upon these cues.

In addition to the semantic, syntactic, and orthographic clues, the braille and large print reader must respond to spatial features. Smooth hand movements maintain spatial orientation for correct interpretation of symbols for braille readers. The interpretation of various type differences affect reading by low vision, print students.

The uniqueness of the process of reading with braille has comprised the bulk of the chapter. It is hoped that the vision specialist will be so familiar with each media that instruction will focus on the commonalities of braille and print. Each is designed to transmit written information so that the blind and low vision student may also have receptive and expressive media for written language.

CHAPTER 5

ASSESSMENT OF READING SKILLS: FACTORS TO CONSIDER IN ASSESSMENT

THE ASSESSMENT of reading skills of visually impaired children is very similar to the assessment of skills for normally sighted children. A major difficulty is that there are few standardized tests which have been adapted into large print or braille. Factors to consider in selecting tests and other assessment measures that are readily available in braille and large print will be discussed in this chapter. The chapter will also include other tests that are adaptable for visually impaired readers but are not available in braille and large print. Teachers may also adapt informal techniques in the diagnosis of reading skills. Most reading diagnosticians would probably prefer to use a combination of these approaches to suit the needs of the particular child. For a listing of the formal measures available the reader is referred to Swallow (1981); Scholl and Schnur (1976); Genshaft, Dare, and O'Malley (1980); Vander Kolk (1981); and Scholl, (1986).

Assessment of the student's level of performance in reading or other communication skills is necessary to develop long range goals and specific objectives leading to an Individual Education Program (IEP) or an instructional strategy. In planning an assessment, it is important to consider the following factors:

1. Who will assess the child.
2. What tests or informal measures will be used.
3. When the child will be assessed.
4. How the results of the assessment will be interpreted.

Who Will Assess the Child

If the teacher administers the assessment, the teacher can observe the particular strategy that the child uses in response to the items on the test.

For example in reading, the teacher can observe if the child is relying on the first letter of the word, syntax, length of the word, shape of the word, etc. in attacking a new word. The teacher can also observe if the child is using prompts or crutches to unlock words such as worn cards, pictures, or unconscious prompts by the teacher.

What Tests or Informal Measures Will Be Used

In a reading evaluation the teacher should be searching for the level at which the child can be successful in identifying words and where the child will need to use word attach skills to identify more difficult words. The teacher needs to find the point at which the child moves from the independent level to the beginning of the frustration level. The teacher needs to be familiar with the tests so that testing can move quickly and that the child's attention is not lost. Visually impaired children generally read much slower than other children so time is of more importance to them in making assessments (Nolan, 1966). For example, rather than taking 20-30 minutes going through the easy levels of an oral paragraph test, such as the Gilmore Oral Paragraphs Test (GOPT), the teacher could get a quicker reference to the reading level of the child by giving a word identification test such as the Wide Range Achievement Test (WRAT). The teacher and student could enter the GOPT at a level which is closer to the student's independent reading level.

When the Child Will Be Assessed

In planning an assessment at the beginning of a school year or an academic period of time, an hour or two should be set aside for mature children and several short periods of time should be set aside for children with short attention spans. Enough time should be set aside for a thorough in-depth assessment in order that:

1. A holistic picture of the child's skills can be obtained.
2. The child's and the teacher's attentions are focused better toward the task at hand.
3. Enough time is needed to identify the child's independent and frustration levels.

How the Results of the Assessment Will be Interpreted

The teacher needs to use as many means as possible to document the responses and the strategies of the child during the test. Notetaking by the teacher is most common. However, having another teacher present may help improve accuracy of these data collected. Video-taping and tape recording sessions are also helpful in going back over the session for a more detailed analysis and for comparing the child's performance across time.

READING SKILLS TO BE ASSESSED

The teacher who is attempting to determine a visually impaired student's achievement level in reading may consider the following skill areas:

1. Letter knowledge
2. Sight word knowledge
3. Word analysis skills
4. Mechanics of reading
5. Comprehension
6. Perceptual skills
7. Cognitive development
8. Intellectual assessment

Each of these skill areas will be examined according to standardized tests which have been adapted to braille and large print, standardized tests which can be adapted by the teacher, or informal techniques which have been found useful in the diagnosis of problems in braille and large print reading. The diagnostician can find a number of other tests which have been transcribed into large print or braille by volunteer transcribers. A number of tests such as the California Achievement Test and the Reading Skills Test have been published in large type by the American Printing House for the Blind. These tests and others can be located through the central catalog of braille and large print publications compiled by the America Printing House for the Blind. The value of using these standardized tests is somewhat limited due to the lack of visually impaired children in the norming groups and to the necessary adaptations in the tests because of the visual impairment.

Letter and Character Knowledge

Letter knowledge is important to the child reading print, while letter and character knowledge are important to the child reading braille. The teacher will want to discover if the student can recognize individual letters and the same letters within words. Character knowledge or familiarity with the 63 single cell combinations and the 189 braille symbols is important to the reader who is reading books transcribed from the American Edition of Standard English Braille. The teacher can informally assess the child's knowledge of the braille letters, contractions, whole word forms, and other braille symbols by checking the child with a list of the embossed symbols.

The Braille Unit Recognition Battery is a special braille test which was designed to measure mastery of the complete literary Grade 2 braille code. The manual for this test is designed to enable the teacher to administer the test items, analyze the results, and plan individual programs for a student of any age. The battery and manual were completed and field-tested by the American Printing House for the Blind.

Sight Word Knowledge

Sight word knowledge is important in braille as well as large print reading. Some formal measures are available in both media for diagnosis of sight word skills of visually impaired children. Successful readers quickly and accurately recognize the most common words. Sight word knowledge is contrasted with the recognition of words through decoding methods or through use of context. Measures of sight word knowledge assess the student's skill level in reading individual words. Formal measures may be found in one of the several overlapping levels of the Brigance Inventory of Basic Skills. The number of correctly read words will yield a grade level equivalent ranging from 1.1 to 6.2. The Brigance is produced in large boldface print, and a tactile adaptation supplement is to be available through the American Printing House for the Blind. The range of the entire battery is pre-kindergarten through Grade 9 and includes subsections that tap each of the communication skills mentioned in this chapter. The several Brigance batteries are directly suitable to use with large print readers and include word lists in each battery. Brigance batteries contain specific written objectives for each skill and level which make them a favorite assessment tool with many teachers.

The Stanford Diagnostic Reading Test contains a word reading subtest in the Red Level which is appropriate for grades 1-3. The 42 item subtest matches words with a picture of the word meaning. It is available from the American Printing House for the Blind only in large print. This test yields normed scores for grade equivalent, stanine, percentile, and scaled scores matched to the student's grade placement.

The Wide Range Achievement Test contains a reading subtest that is a word recognition test. This brief individually administered achievement test is for grades 1-6 in Level 1 and grades 7-12 in Level 2. Scores are translated into grade equivalents and both levels have been prepared in large print and braille by the American Printing House for the Blind. The results from this test could confirm the results from other related reading tests. Its major value would be to give the diagnostician levels of reading comprehension, arithmetic, comprehension and spelling for the visually impaired child.

Although unavailable in braille, a number of individual diagnostic reading tests can be transcribed into braille for use with blind children. Many of these tests have word recognition sections which can be used quite readily although the time limits and norms for sighted children are not applicable. Among the more popularly used tests are the Botel Reading Inventory, the Diagnostic Reading Scales, the Durrell Analysis of Reading Difficulty, and the Gates-McKilliop Reading Diagnostic Tests. The Diagnostic Reading Scales is not currently available in braille or large print, but the scores it provides compare closely to the scores obtained with other tests in braille and large print including the Stanford Achievement Tests and the Gilmore Oral Reading Test.

The authors have found that the grade equivalent scores derived from the use of the word lists of the Diagnostic Reading Scales correspond with the suggested readability level of many series produced in braille and large print. The three graded word lists have overlapping grade equivalencies, ranging from 1.1 to 6.5 graded reading levels. The lists are especially useful to obtain a quick estimate of the student's reading level so that more in-depth testing materials may be selected and testing times may be used more efficiently. Two popular achievement tests having word recognition sections are the Woodcock-Johnson Psychoeducational Battery and the Peabody Individual Achievement Test.

In addition to the normed referenced tests described above, the teacher may use informal measures to quickly identify the student's recognition of the most common words. The Dolch Basic Sight Word List is one of the most popular lists used by publishers in designing reading series and formal tests. Although based on studies of word frequencies that were conducted in the 1930s, the content of the list is still applicable. The words may be divided into five levels, preprimer through third grade, and used to assess the student's sight word knowledge. The teacher may obtain a percent of correctly identified sight words at each of the five levels. The Dolch words are available on individual cards from the American Printing House for the Blind in braille and large print. An update of the Dolch list has been compiled by Johnson (1971) on the basis of more recent word frequency studies.

More important to day-to-day reading may be the student's knowledge of the most common words in the current basal reader. The teacher may use the list of vocabulary words printed in the back of most basal readers to test the student's mastery of the vocabulary of that book in isolation. The vocabulary may be printed or brailled on cards or in lists and presented to the child individually. The teacher may obtain a percentage of correctly read words by dividing the number of words read correctly by the number of words attempted. The words missed may become the target words for subsequent instruction.

Publishers of basal reading series frequently provide tests in the teaching manual or separately prepared publications that will assist the teacher in identifying the sight word identification level of the student using the vocabulary that has been introduced in the reader to date. Several of the reading series which are currently produced by the American Printing House for the Blind in braille and large print contain vocabulary tests and suggestions for reteaching. The PATTERNS reading series, the series that is written for the sequential introduction of the braille code, includes word recognition tests at every level.

In noting the student's reading of sight words, the teacher may record the student's actual errors as well as correct responses. By analyzing the student's errors, the teacher may determine the types of errors that the student is making. If, for example, the student reads "who" for "what" the teacher may include both words in the pool of words to be learned since the student may only really recognize either word as a sight word when both of them are learned.

The list of vocabulary words included in a book may be used to predict the student's reading ability in a particular book and may be useful in selecting a book. An accuracy of at least 75% in reading the isolated vocabulary of a book is recommended for students reading independent of teacher assistance. Accuracy between 50% and 75% is acceptable for reading with teacher assistance.

Word Analysis Skills

Word analysis skills include the phonic skills which are used to analyze the correspondence between the letters and the sounds of a word. Such a relationship may be referred to as a graphophoneme relationship or a sound-symbol correspondence. Teacher's manuals and tests may use terms such as phonics, word study, or word analysis to refer to the student's skills in using consonant and vowel patterns to identify a word.

Another word analysis skill, structural analysis, enables a student to read unfamiliar words that are made up of familiar words and syllables. Beginning readers are using structural analysis when they read "helped" by recognizing the root word "help" to which the inflected ending "ed" has been added. Experienced readers use structural analysis to identify words using prefixes, suffixes, and root words. Word analysis skills may also be referred to as synthesis because the sound of the word is identified by building on the letters and syllables.

The visually impaired student needs to be especially efficient in word analysis skills. The reader of braille (Nolan & Kederis, 1969) or large print is probably reading words by single cells or clusters of letters. Therefore, the visually impaired reader must continually synthesize words in reading. A formal assessment of the word analysis skills of braille and large print readers may be obtained with the Stanford Achievement Test Word-Study Skills subtests. Forms E and F have been adapted into braille and large print by the American Printing House for the Blind. The Primary Level 2 for grades 2.5 to 3.4 through the Intermediate Level 2 grades 5.5 to 6.9 include Word Study Skills tests. Items at the Primary Level 2 include 64 multiple choice items divided into a part on beginning and ending sounds and a part on visual phonics. The print form of the Stanford Achievemet Test was modified by adapting the directions for administering the test (Morris, 1974). Although time limits are not required, suggested time limits were expanded to two and one-half times the time limit for normally seeing children for braille readers and one and one-half for large print readers. The norms for seeing children should be used with caution for this section of the test.

The Standard Diagnostic Reading Test, available in braille and large print from the American Printing House for the Blind, is in four levels: Red (1-3), Green (3-5), Brown (5-8), and Blue (9-12). The first level of the test, Red (1-3), is highly pictorial and is available only in large print. Each level of the test includes a phonetic analysis subtest and provides normed scores by grade level. Levels beyond the first level include a test in structural analysis with two parts—word division and blending.

A formal test of oral reading accuracy, comprehension, and speed that is commercially available in braille and large print is the Gilmore Oral Paragraphs Test. This test has been reported in research studies with blind children (Harley & Rawls, 1969; Henderson, 1973; Truan, 1978). The pupil is asked to read short graded passages orally while the administrator clocks the speed and marks a copy of the test according to types of error. Questions are asked at the end of each passage to measure comprehension. Accuracy, rate, and comprehension scores are normed so that a grade level equivalent can be obtained for each score. The test is short and easy to administer with norms for sighted children, but norms for blind children are not yet available. Two forms (C and D) of the test have been copied into braille for use with visually impaired readers by the American Printing House for the Blind. The test is useful for analyzing the types of oral reading errors such as repetitions, omissions, substitutions, etc. However, care should be used in interpretation of results. Although silent and oral reading is very similar for beginning readers through the first primary year, there is little evidence to indicate much similarity between the two processes after readers begin to obtain proficiency in silent reading (Spache, 1976).

Word analysis skills can also be determined by interpreting individual diagnostic reading tests which are not published in braille. These tests include the Botel Reading Inventory, Durrell Analysis of Reading Difficulty, Gates-McKillop Reading Diagnostic Tests, Diagnostic Reading Scales, and the Peabody Individual Achievement Test. Although these instruments can be transcribed into braille for the blind reader, caution should be used in interpreting the results since the tests were not standardized with blind children.

Word analysis skills can be further pinpointed through an examination of the child's errors with an Informal Reading Inventory (IRI) (Betts, 1967; Fry, 1972; and Aulls, 1982). It may be used to assess word recognition accuracy, comprehension, and reading speed. These teacher-constructed inventories are designed to provide the best possible match between the student's reading skills and the actual reading materials that will be used. This matching between the materials and skills can also be obtained by using formal reading measures described earlier in this chapter. The advantage of using the informal reading inventory is that the actual reading materials are used.

An informal inventory usually consists of a series of passages chosen from a book, estimated to be at the child's reading level and teacher-made comprehension questions. Typical passages may be taken from a basal series or from other textbooks. Each passage is approximately 50 to 300 words long, depending on the reading level. Two passages may be prepared for each level, one for oral and one for silent reading beyond the second grade level. As the student reads orally, the teacher makes notes on a copy of the passage from the child's reader.

A suggested marking system for recording a student's oral reading is show in Figure 14. This marking system may be used to obtain the accuracy, comprehension, and rate scores in the IRI and for analysis of the reading miscues. All miscues are recorded including those counted and to counted as errors. Errors include insertions, omissions, repetitions, mispronunciations or substitutions, and teacher prompts. Responses not counted as errors include spelling words, self-corrections, multiple attempts, hesitations or frustrations, and ignored punctuation.

Marking Symbols for an IRI

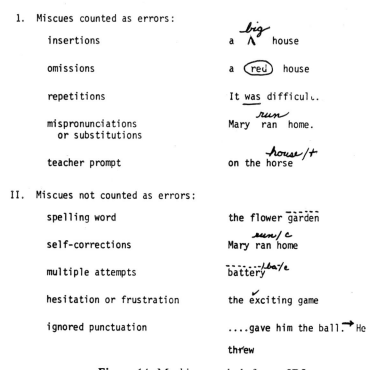

Figure 14. Marking symbols for an IRI.

The oral reading errors in each passage are tallied and a percentage of accuracy is obtained. Upon completion of the oral reading, comprehension questions are answered. The teacher may prepare questions requiring both literal and inferential answers and may include questions about vocabulary meaning, sequence, and main idea. A percentage of comprehension can be obtained by comparing correct answers to the number of questions, and a rate of reading may be derived by dividing the actual number of words read by the time in minutes. For older students, the teacher may wish to prepare a comparable reading passage to be read silently for comparison of oral and silent reading comprehension and speed. In addition to scores, the teacher will have a pool of reading errors to examine for an error pattern.

Goodman (1973) expanded the informal reading inventory in a technique they called miscue analysis for analyzing the quality of mistakes of print readers called "miscues." The technique may be applied to readers of large print or braille using information obtained with an Informal Reading Inventory. Working under the psycholinguistic assumption that reading errors were not made at random, Goodman (1973) defined any discrepancy between the print text and the student's oral reading as a miscue. The term was chosen to emphasize the interaction between the reader and the three redundant cueing systems of English: orthography (letter sound relationship), syntax (predictive word order), and semantics (overall passage meaning). The reader has available each of these three sources of information to identify an unfamiliar word by making a logical prediction. A specific plan for remediation follows directly from the analysis of the child's reading weaknesses and, more important, strengths. The key is in the system of collecting and tabulating the child's oral reading errors or miscues. All miscues are not equal; some are irrelevant and some are very good signs of potential reading success. Even the most fluent adult reader of print or braille will make miscues when reading orally.

Information obtained from the child's performance on several IRI passages of different difficulty can be used to determine three performance levels: independent, instructional, and frustration. The exact percentage of word recognition and comprehension accuracy used as a criteria for each level differs slightly among authors of reading texts (Betts, 1967; Fortell, 1985; Fry, 1972), but a general guide would include:

Independent Level:　　word recognition accuracy　　95 to 100%

　　　　　　　　　　　comprehension　　　　　　　　90 to 100%

The level at which the child can read with relative ease and independence is the level at which the child can read library books or other material without assistance. There is little in the material that the student cannot manage independently. The teacher may obtain a quick estimate of the reading level by having the student read orally and determining that the student made no more than one error per 20 words. This quick estimate technique is especially useful in selecting recreational reading, for example, in checking out books from the library.

Instructional Level: word recognition and accuracy   90 to 94%

                        comprehension   75 to 90%

The instructional level is the level at which the student will normally receive reading instruction. The student should know most of the words, but not all of the words in the passage.

Frustration Level: word recognition and accuracy   89% or less

                        comprehension   50% or less

At the frustration level, the material is too difficult for the student. Consistent presentation of material at this level in which there are too many unfamiliar words inhibits reading progress and may result in persistent reading problems.

An example of the information obtained from an informal reading inventory might reveal that a student's reading levels are:

        Independent Level: second grade, second half

        Instructional Level: third grade, first half

        Frustration Level: fourth grade

Figure 15 is a sample of a passage that has been marked with the error symbol system. Also included are comprehension questions and a tally of results.

An informal reading assessment chart can be useful in comparing a student's performance from time to time. Keeping a chart for each reader can be very useful in the measurement of progress and the assessment of reading problems. Other sources of reading data can be included on this chart, such as the student's accuracy in reading individual vocabulary words in the reading book and graded word lists such as the Dolch Word List.

An analysis of errors over one or several passages may reveal a pattern for similar errors. The student might rely consistently on initial consonant sounds to the exclusion of other cues. Perhaps the reader predicts words from context too quickly or misses words because of perceptual reversals, undeveloped decoding skills, or a limited knowledge of the braille code. Although the same errors may not be consistently repeated, an error analysis should reveal a pattern which can alert the teacher to the child's weaknesses in word identification skills.

Mother waves good-by to Father each morning. She begins the ^(to/c)

housework soon after he leaves. Bob and Jane help her before they ^(s)

go to school. They dry ^(dr-ḷ⁺·/c) the dishes and clean their own ^(---/c) rooms. After → From/c

Mother has finished ^(---/c) the work indooors, she goes out to her pretty ^(v/c)

flower garden. ^(v/⁺/c) She tends ^(ten/----/c ✓) it nearly ^(ever) every day for about an hour.

Mother does all her work with ^(of/c) great care.

✓ 1. What does Mother do as Father is leaving?

✓ 2. What does Mother do after Father has gone?

✓ 3. When do Bob and Jane help Mother?

✓ 4. Where does Mother go after she has finished the work indoors?

✓ 5. How long does she work in her garden each day?

% Comprehension Questions Correct 100%.

Words Read 67

Errors 4

% Words Read Correctly 94%.

Time 2 min. 35 sec.

Reading Rate 27 words per min.

Student Jimmy S.

Date 1/8/--

Passage Difficulty fourth grade

Figure 15. Sample of marking and scoring an IRI.

The use of several word identification skills may be required for some words. The reader who depends on one or two strategies, may miss the necessary cue to identify the word and make an error. When this is a consistent problem, it points up a need for instruction in specific word identification skills. The following examples of Common Reading Errors shows many error types. Some errors are common to readers of any mode and some are peculiar to braille.

COMMON READING ERRORS

Actual Phrase	Response Phrase	Word identification Strategy — ERROR
Errors Common To All Readers		
I can *hold*	I can *help*	Use of initial consonant only
the big *cap*	the big *cup*	Use of initial and final consonant but confusion of medial vowel
is *making*	is *running*	Reliance on end of the word
they took	they looked	Use of middle of word
spend money	*send* money	Missed initial blend
for the *gardiner*	for the *garden*	Word ending omitted
the *baby* bed	the *baby's* bed	Word ending added
Jim *asked*	Jim *said*	Reliance on sentence meaning
a *circus* monkey	a *trained* monkey	Reliance on passage meaning
the new *grill*	the new *girl*	Use of configuration, and initial and final consonant
Errors Common To Braille Readers		
for *more*	for *us*	Vertical braille reversal
to hear *of*	to hear *with*	Horizontal braille reversal
He can *do*	He can *have*	Diagonal braille reversal
is *blind*	is *below*	Vertical alignment
a *little*	*all*	Horizontal alignment
of *these* good things	of *their* good things	Missed dot
It is *not*	it is *you*	Added dot
They *played*	they *play*	Word ending
to the fort	*from* the fort	Spacing and vertical alignment
His mother	*Here* mother	Vertical alignment error and confusion of capital dot with dot 5
Some of your	*So with* you	Missed dot in first of sentence and changed subsequent words to fit sentence pattern.

Figure 16. Common reading errors.

After initial assessments of reading skills, shorter progress probes are helpful to the teacher in making judgments concerning mastery levels attained by her students. Curriculum-based assessment is an evaluation procedure in which teachers can routinely modify a student's instructional program. Some simple curriculum-based instruction measures in reading include supplying words deleted from the text, saying the meanings of underlined words in the text and reading aloud from word lists or text passages. The teacher records the words read correctly in one minute. For example, the student may read 22 words correctly per minute on a primer level selection and 35 words per minute at the end of the first grade reader. Results of studies show that such curriculum-based measures are highly correlated with performance on standardized and norm-referenced tests (Deno, 1985). Advantages of these curriculum-based instruction measures have been low cost, high reliability and validity, simplicity, and ease of understanding by parents, teachers and students.

Mechanics of Reading

Braille readers may be penalized by using their fingers and hands in a manner which slows the reading process. Excessive up and down movements, undue pressure on the fingertips, incorrect use of the hands in finding the next line, and many other factors related to mechanics of reading can cause reading problems for blind children. A checklist in Appendix D can be used by the teacher to diagnose problems in reading mechanics. Similarly, poor posture, incorrect position of the book, glare in lighting, or irregular eye movements in tracking can also cause problems for the low vision print reader. Assistance in diagnosing these problems can be found in *Understanding Low Vision* by Randall Jose (1983).

Comprehension

Reading comprehension can be determined through the use of the braille or large print forms of the paragraph meaning section of the Stanford Achievement Test. This test consists of a series of graduated paragraphs which contain one or more omitted words. The student must demonstrate comprehension of the paragraph by selecting from four choices a word to fill each blank. The test purports to provide a functional measure of the pupil's ability to comprehend connected discourse ranging in length from single sentences to paragraphs of several sentences. Comprehension levels vary from extremely simple recognition to the making of inferences from several related sentences.

Reading comprehension can also be determined through the use of the paragraph reading test of the Durrell Listening-Reading Series. This test has been validated through a field evaluation with 65 braille subjects from reading levels 1-3. The Durrell is designed to provide a comparison of children's reading and listening abilities. The series consists of tests in both listening and reading at primary, intermediate, and advanced grades. In the primary tests, the student is required to classify a statement under a category. In the upper levels, the test items vary in difficulty from simple factual recall to inference, classification, and other types of interpretation. No attempt is made to analyze types of mental processes in relation to reading and listening. Suggestions for assisting low achieving readers given in the manual are based on test scores. The unique feature of this test is the comparison of listening and reading skills. The Durrell Listening-Reading Series is available in braille and large print from the American Printing House for the Blind.

Students reading at a first grade level beyond the preprimer stage should be able to use the Durrell (Morris, 1976). However, practice materials may be needed for marking answer choices. The vocabulary test requires that the child relate a word to one of three categories in a cluster at the primary level. The category words which constitute the options in each cluster are explained by the teacher in both the listening and reading tests. Words have been adapted for the blind reader in place of pictures for use in column headings. This procedure places blind readers at some disadvantage because they must read the option words without the help of a picture. With this understanding, the test norms for the print edition can be used with the braille reader.

The Gilmore Oral Reading Test, available in braille and large print, is a test used largely for accuracy and rate of oral reading (see Word Analysis Skills). It also can be used to measure comprehension. However, the comprehension questions follow a repetitive pattern which makes it sometimes easy to guess the correct answers.

Several standardized tests permit the comparative study of content vocabularies such as the Diagnostic Vocabulary Test (Committee on Diagnostic Reading Tests) and the California Reading Test (California Test Bureau). The vocabulary sections of intelligence tests such as the Standford-Binet and Weschler Intelligence Scale for Children-Revised could also provide a quick screening method for determining the vocabulary performance of children.

Comprehension skills can also be determined through an IRI or through other print reading tests which can be transcribed into braille. These tests include the Durrell Analysis of Reading Difficulty, Gates-McKillop Reading Diagnostic Tests, Botel Reading Inventory, and Diagnostic Reading Scales.

Perceptual Skills

Auditory perceptual ability is closely related to success in reading. The measurement of auditory discrimination, auditory sequencing ability, auditory separation, auditory blending, auditory clozure, and other auditory perceptual skills is discussed in the chapter on the Teaching of Listening skills.

A knowledge of the child's visual acuity and field of vision can be helpful in the diagnosis of reading problems. However, a functional evaluation of the child's ability to use vision is much more meaningful in planning a reading program. Some scales which have been designed specifically for low vision children are the Visual Efficiency Scale (Barraga, 1970), the Diagnostic Assessment Procedure (DAP) (Barraga & Morris, 1980) and the Functional Vision Inventory (Langley, 1980).

The DAP scale is a criterion-referenced instrument based on the assumptions that effective use of vision is learned and that visual functioning and perceptual-cognitive development are interrelated. The DAP scale is designed to determine information about the low vision learner's visual function from birth to beginning discrimination of print symbols. The items on the scale are especially suitable for the assessment of visual perceptual skills which are needed in reading print. A strength of the DAP is the matching sequence of planned visual learning lessons organized into eight categories of visual developmental milestones and written so that they can easily be translated into an individual educational program for the child. Another advantage of the DAP is that the items are designed to be viewed by low vision children. A weakness of the DAP is that the scale contains few items at the birth to 2-year level.

For low functioning children, a more appropriate instrument is the Functional Vision Inventory (Langley, 1980). The Functional Vision Inventory was designed primarily for multiply handicapped low vision children. The scale provides assessment data in such areas as structural defects, reflexive reactions, eye movement, near and distance vision, visual field, and visual perception. A strength of the Functional Vision Inventory is the matching of training activities in important visual perceptual skills such as fixation, tracking, scanning, eye-hand integration, and form, shape, and color discrimination. Another strength is that the scale starts at a very low level of visual perceptual functioning and contains appropriate for low functioning children. This scale makes extensive use of penlights and colorful toys which can be used to keep the attention of the children during the administration.

Visual perceptual tests used with normally seeing children can sometimes be used with low vision children if they have the visual acuity and field to see the figures. These tests of visual perceptual abilities which include tests for such areas as visual motor, visual memory, and visual discrimination are The Bender Visual Motor Gestalt, the Frostig Developmental Test of Visual Perception, and the Visual-Motor Integration Test. The Motor-Free Visual Perception Test is a test which avoids motor involvement and can be used to assess overall visual perceptual processing ability of children.

The visual functioning of the low vision child may also be assessed by informal observational techniques. For example, the distance that the child uses to see details in a picture gives some indication of visual acuity. The ability to match objects and shapes may indicate ability to discriminate between visual and perceptual ability. An observation checklist on the DAP could be very helpful in making this informal assessment.

Selecting the reading medium is an important consideration for the low vision student. When the first classes for partially seeing children were initiated in the early part of this century, teachers were trained to use techniques which would save the sight of their children. Children with large amounts of residual vision were taught to read braille in order to conserve vision. In recent years, emphasis has been placed on "sight-utilization" rather than "sight-saving." Research studies by Barraga (1964) and Ashcroft, Halliday, and Barraga (1965) have shown that many low vision children who were reading braille could be taught to read print materials after a period of visual perceptual training.

Low vision students may read both print and braille in their educational programs. Some children may read signs and labels in print, but read books and lengthy publications in braille. Some children may read history and literature in braille, but prefer to do their arithmetic in print. The visually impaired student who is beginning to learn to read may be able to learn to read using several media stimultaneously including large print, braille, print on a closed circuit television or computer monitor, paperless braille, or Optacon. Other visually impaired students may not be cognitively or perceptually able to interrelate several symboling systems. Low vision students with the potential learning problems described in Chapter 7 may have the most difficulty integrating print and braille. If reading instruction is continued in both modes for these students, progress can be slow. Instruction in reading with focus on a single medium may assist in solving this problem. Certain factors should be considered in order to make the decision about a student's primary reading medium:

1. Prognosis of eye condition
2. Visual acuity
3. Visual field
4. Focal distance
5. Type size required
6. Reading rate
7. Visual stamina
8. Probable need
9. Basic mode of function
10. Attitude of child and parents

Prognosis of Eye Condition

Children with certain kinds of unstable eye conditions may not be able to continue in print through their school career. Progressive myopia, retinitis pigmentosa, congenital glaucoma, and retinoblastoma are examples of eye conditions in which loss of vision can be progressive. The instruction in braille may be provided when the student's vision deteriorates so that print reading is not efficient.

Visual Acuity

The use of visual acuity obtained by the doctor is a starting point for the teacher in choosing a reading medium. The most useful reports contain both distance and near acuity with and without corrective lenses. The teacher will want to confirm the near acuities with a variety of classroom materials. Procedures for obtaining visual acuity may be found in *Visual Impairments in the Schools* (Harley & Lawrence, 1984).

Visual Field

The child with a visual field limited to no more than three letters in print may only be able to read print at a very slow rate. Print reading may be useful for reading labels and signs, but volume reading would be laborious. The visual field can be detected in an eye examination by a perimeter or tangent screen. The teacher could estimate the visual field or visual span in reading by informal techniques or by using the perimeter accessory to binocular testing instruments, such as the Keystone Telebinocular.

Focal Distance

The focal distance or the distance between the reading material and the student's eyes may be determined by observation with a tape measure. The standard distance of 16 inches may be too great for some low vision students. If the student must move to less than 3 inches from the reading material to read, reading may become physically exhausting.

Type Size Required

Type sizes of printed material are measured in points with 72 points corresponding to 1 inch. Standard large print is 18 point type or one-fourth inch in height. The type in "large print" books may very somewhat if the book has been photo-enlarged. The final type size will depend on the type size and style of the original print copy. Individual differences among low vision children indicate requirements of type sizes ranging from 12 points to 24 or 30 points. If the child must read 24 to 30 point type, there will be a limited quantity of available material. Optical aids can help make print accessible. An examination by a low vision specialist, who may prescribe an appropriate optical aid, is a first step in learning to make use of an optical aid.

Reading Rate

If the beginning reader is reading large print at an excessively slow rate (10 words per minute) after a sufficient trial, the emphasis on print reading may be unwarranted. The mean rates for large print readers in grades 4-6 on content level materials of science, social studies, and literature has been measured at 79 words per minute compared to 59 words per minute for braille students with the same passages. Normally sighted reading rates were 179 words per minute. At the high school level large print students averaged 95 words per minute on content material, braille readers averaged 83, and normally sighted readers averaged 215 words per minute. Braille readers take 2 to 3 times as much time and large print readers from 2.3 to 2.6 times as much time to read the same material (Nolan, 1966).

Visual Stamina

If the child tires easily from print reading, tactual reading should also be considered. The teacher should be alert to signs of fatigue such as headaches, watery eyes, neck and shoulder strain, and other physical signs of stress. Use of adjustable reading stands, optical aids, adjustable height desks and chairs may help increase visual stamina.

Probable Need

Research has shown that mentally retarded children as a group do very poorly in braille. Nolan and Kederis (1969) found evidence that suggested that students with an intelligence quotient below 85 find braille to be an extremely inefficient medium of communication. Adults or adventitiously blinded youth may find braille to be difficult to learn, especially when residual vision is sufficient to continue a limited amount of print reading. Listening can often be substituted for print in gaining information at a faster rate.

Primary Mode of Function

Informal observation by the teacher can be used to determine if the child is primarily functioning visually or tactally in the exploration of the environment. The teacher may place several interesting objects for the child to explore and observe whether the child uses eyes and/or hands. A child's primary mode of functioning should be considered in determining reading mode.

Attitude of Child and Parents

The school environment certainly seems to make a big difference in attitudes toward print and braille. For example, a much higher percentage of low vision children in public day schools use print then in residential schools for the blind. Sighted parents may prefer print while blind parents may prefer braille for their low vision children. The child's attitude will be a large factor in the selection of the reading medium emphasis. It is much easier to teach braille to children or youth who have accepted their blindness. Experienced teachers can attest to the fact that it is almost impossible to develop good braille readers with pupils who avoid any symbol which associates them with blindness.

Tactual Perception

In the diagnosis of reading problems of the blind reader, special attention should be given to tactual perception. The Roughness Discrimination Test is a test of tactual perception. This test was designed primarily to evaluate readiness to begin braille reading. It consists of sets of squares of sandpaper of different degrees of coarseness. The child is required to indicate which of four squares is different from the others. It is recommended that this test be given to students at the kindergarten or first grade level prior to any attempt to begin braille instruction.

Predictive validity of the test was determined by correlating 156 Roughness Discrimination Test scores at the beginning of the year with reading criteria at the end of the same school year. Concurrent validity was found by correlating test scores and reading criteria at the same sitting. A problem with this test is that tactual sensitivity is not the only factor relevant to braille reading. Roughness discrimination does not measure tactual perception of shape, size, or direction discrimination ability of embossed designs.

Although not a test, *Touch and Tell,* a book in three volumes by the American Printing House for the Blind (Duncan, 1969) can be very helpful in making an informal assessment of the child's tactual discrimination ability. This book which is designed to meet the tactual reading readiness needs for young blind children, consists of embossed geometric designs and braille dots that are graduated in size to provide for gross to fine tactual discrimination skills. *Modern Methods of Teaching Braille,* which provides a graduated series of tactual patterns, could be used to assess tactual discrimination by having the pupil sample sections of the book (Stocker, 1970). The criterion-referenced tests of the Mangold Developmental Program of Tactile Perception and Braille Recognition could also be used to measure tactile recognition.

Mommers (1976) reported research to standardize braille reading tests for use in elementary schools in Holland. Subjects included the total blind school-age population of children in Holland, which numbered 120 children between the ages of 6 and 15. The study investigated the relationship between reading achievement and residual vision, hand movement during reading, verbal intelligence, and perception. The amount or residual vision bore little relationship to reading ability of blind children but the way children moved their hands during reading bore a strong relationship. Mommers concluded that the best readers have an even flow of hand movement, light pressure, and relaxed hand muscles when learning to read braille books. The most interesting part of his study indicated that, of all the various haptic measures used, form discrimination and figure orientation were more important than size and roughness discrimination. This finding is important to reading readiness problems because blind children need to be exposed to materials which are designed to teach discrimination of form and figure more than size and roughness.

Cognitive Development

Children who have difficulty acquiring spatial concepts such as right, left, over, under may later have difficulty in academic tasks that involve spatial and sequential concepts. These students may have trouble locating the beginning of the page in reading or have difficulty following teacher directions. Such problems may be detected by several tests of the visually impaired child's concepts of spatial and positional concepts.

The Tactile Test of Basic Concepts (TTBC) (Caton, 1977) was designed to be a tactual analog of the Boehm Test of Basic Concepts which was designed for normally sighted children (See Figure 17). The Boehm test is useful with many low vision students since it uses bold illustrations. Both the TTBC and the Boehm consist of 50 items designed to assess the child's understanding of space (location, direction, orientation, and dimensions), time, and quantity in a two-dimensional format. The TTBC achieves a tactile representation of the printed Boehm test by using plastic sheets and the basic geometric forms comparable to the original print test. Acceptable reliability and content validity may be questioned for normally sighted children with the Boehm Test of Basic Concepts and for blind children with the Tactile Test of Basic Concepts. Whether the mastery of the concepts is related to achievement in the first years of school may also be questioned. Although these tests were not designed particularly for reading readiness, the concepts of "top," "over," "back," etc. could be useful for teachers giving directions concerning orientation to braille reading and writing tasks.

The Hill Performance Test of Selected Positional Concepts (Hill, 1981) was found to be valid and reliable with 273 visually impaired 6-10 year olds. This test, designed primarily for evaluating concepts needed in orientation and mobility, could also provide useful information on concepts needed in reading. Children are asked to demonstrate concepts by identifying various positional relationships of body parts and by moving the body and objects in relationship to other objects.

The Body-Image of Blind Children by Cratty and Sams (1968) has a body-image training scale which can be used to evaluate concepts related to various types of body movement. This scale, like the Hill Performance Test, contains many concepts which could be useful in reading.

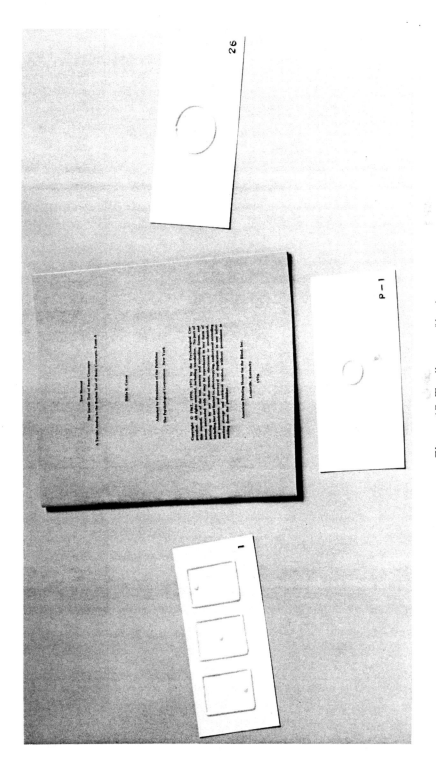

Figure 17. Tactile test of basic concepts.

Intellectual Assessment

Most intelligence tests used with the visually impaired rely heavily on verbal sections of the tests. Examples of such tests are the Perkins-Binet and the Wechsler Intelligence Scale for Children-Revised (WISC). The verbal sections of the intelligence tests may be quite useful in the diagnosis of reading problems but the performance tests will probably provide little additional information.

The Perkins-Binet is an adaptation of the 1960 Stanford-Binet. In addition to the verbal sections, the Perkins-Binet has some performance items at the lower age levels of the test. There are some performance measures of intelligence which have been used with adults, such as the Haptic-Intelligence Scale (an adaptation of the Wechsler Adult Intelligence Scale (WAIS), the Stanford-Kohs Block Design Test, and the Blind Learning Aptitude Test (BLAT), but these tests have not proved useful with young school-age children.

The Wechsler Intelligence Scale for Children-Revised (WISCR) and its preschool counterpart, the Wechsler Preschool and Primary Scale of Intelligence (WPPSI), have become almost standard instruments for individual testing in schools. The five verbal tests which have not been adapted are: information, comprehension, arithmetic, similarities, and vocabulary. They may be used with visually impaired children. The performance scale may be used with some low vision children, but the score should be reported separately because of its heavy visual orientation. Test administration is essentially the same with blind and sighted persons, and the norms for sighted children may be used, although some of the items are inappropriate for blind children. The lack of a performance test for the blind is the major shortcoming of these tests. Since the WISC-R and the Binet are tests reserved for use by a psychologist, the vision teacher will be more familiar with the reports rather than the procedures for administering the test.

The Wechsler Preschool and Primary Scale of Intelligence (WPPSI) test was developed as a downward extension of the WISC (4.2 to 6.6 years). The test is limited in use with blind children because visual experience is needed with many of the items. It is also not very useful as a reading diagnostic tool since it was not designed for blind preschool children.

The Slosson Intelligence Test for Children and Adults has been administered orally with visually impaired children as a verbal measure of intelligence (Harley & Rawls, 1970). This test is a individually administered measure with the purpose of serving as a screening instrument in the evaluation of mental ability. The test has been criticized for lacking specificity in the norming sample and its large and variable standard deviation (Salvia & Ysseldyke, 1981).

SETTING GOALS AND OBJECTIVES

Frequently, teachers of large print and braille reading are confronted with students who have significant reading needs. The range and depth of these needs are often mammoth at first glance and the immediacy of the situation suggests instruction through every appropriate method and material. The teacher may initiate instruction including many techniques: phonics, structural analysis, sight word identification, utilization of context clues, tactual discrimination, braille character recognition, etc. This "shotgun" approach to the reading instructional attempts to remediate all deficiencies at the same time, may prove ineffective. Some reading instructional pellets may not hit the target, wasting the effort of both teacher and student. When the target is hit without the full force of the instructional shot, the problems may not be eliminated. Therefore, the logical initial step in planning braille reading instruction is to carefully locate the student's reading needs and to aim instruction at these areas.

A systematic plan of instruction and a concise method for recording student progress is essential for the teaching of reading to visually impaired students. Such written planning and reporting must be concise or the teacher can become bogged down with many lesson plans, evaluations, grade cards, and final reports. A system in which plans and lesson objectives grow from evaluation can result in a cycle of test-teach-test with continual monitoring of student progress.

There are three basic reasons for developing written instructional plans. First, the teacher may be responsible for the reading instruction of several students, all working at varying levels and receiving individualized instruction. Without written objectives for each student, the many small related objectives leading to reading become too complex for the teacher to remember. Secondly, evaluations are a means of communication to other teachers and parents of the student's strengths and needs through the documenting of each student's progress. Legal requirements for an Individual Educational Program (IEP) play a third role in written instructional plans. Legislation, such as P.L. 94-142, coupled with state legislation and local guidelines, has greatly increased the necessity for teachers to plan and to record student progress. Such requirements provide a structural framework for preparing reports. Knowing the essential components required in preparing written plans for each child can speed the process of reporting.

Instructional planning is based on evalation and necessitates a knowledge of the child's strengths and needs obtained through diagnosis. Any plans should include a statement of the child's level of performance. Information will be available to many teachers about the student's previous work with grade and testing, such as achievement tests and psychological evaluation. A written statement is required of the student's present level of performance that identifies strengths and need. General tips for wording the results of an educational evaluation are contained in Appendix E, Writing Tips for Reporting an Educational Assessment. The teacher may need to conduct additional evaluations for selection of materials and targeting specific objectives. A report may include an extensive compilation of evaluative diagnostic information to assist in instructional planning. Ultimately, a concise summative statement is needed. Such a statement of reading performance for an elementary-level braille reader might include:

> "Jeff's overall reading performance is at a mid-fourth grade level. His strongest skills are in oral and silent reading comprehension and word meaning, which rated at a mid-fifth grade level. He is less successful with using word identification skills of phonics and structural analysis, which are rated at an early fourth grade level."

From the result of evaluative data, the teacher sets goals. These goals are basically of two types. Long-term goals define the goal for the whole year. Through setting long-range goals, the teacher makes realistic and purposeful plans for the year. An example of a long-range goal for a braille reader experiencing difficulty in reading might be:

> "By the end of the year, Sue will have increased her reading skills so that she will be able to successfully read at a fifth grade level."

Short-term goals are the specific step-by-step objectives by which the student will achieve the year-end goal. Examples of short-term objectives for braille readers in rate and mechanics are:

> "To increase George's braille reading rate and efficiency, he will orally read a passage from the current basal at least five words per minute faster than previously measured and maintain the level of accuracy and comprehension with an informal reading inventory procedure."
> "Ann will increase her use of good braille reading mechanics to include light, even finger pressure and raised wrist as measured on the Mechanics of Reading checklist."

Legal requirements of an IEP necessitate an additional description of any educational services which a student receives outside the regular classroom. Since the vision teachers may be responsible for such service, they should include information related to reading instruction which includes:

1. The identification of specific services;
2. An indication of the extent to which the child will be able to participate in the regular school program;
3. A notation of the schedule of services to be provided and the beginning date and targeted date for mastery;
4. The justification for placement;
5. A list of individuals responsible for implementing the instruction.

Educational planning should be a continuing cycle of evaluation-planning-teaching-evaluating. As such, it will have built-in, periodic re-evaluations and identification of new objectives.

SUMMARY

The tests and scales which have been described are illustrative of the types of tests which could be used in an assessment of a visually impaired child. There are many other instruments which could be adapted for use with these children. Perhaps, the experienced teacher may want to use some informal procedures and techniques which come from training materials, books, and experience in assessment. These selected instruments could be very helpful in providing useful information on a child who is new to the class or to provide some objective information to confirm the clinical judgment of the experienced teacher. Some teachers may know from the results of these tests how to plan a remedial program for the child. The manuals of the assessment instruments are often very useful in providing suggestions for how to use the information to plan individual programs. With experience, using trial and error, the teacher or diagnostician will soon learn to choose a favorite battery of tests which provide the kind of information needed to plan the most effective reading program.

The information from the diagnostic evaluation should be used to plan an individual reading program which includes a systematic plan of instruction based upon carefully planned goals and objectives and which includes plans for monitoring and evaluation. Maintaining an appropriate reading environment through evaluation-instruction-re-evaluation is the best plan for providing a successful reading program for each visually impaired student.

CHAPTER 6

IDENTIFYING VISUALLY IMPAIRED STUDENTS WITH LEARNING PROBLEMS

PREVIOUS CHAPTERS have described the specialized and adapted instruction that is necessary to help visually impaired students develop oral and written communication skills. The purpose of this chapter is to identify the characteristics of visually impaired students who are having difficulty meeting their potential in reading and writing even with the specialized adaptations outline in Chapters 2-5. For whatever reason, such visually impaired students do not learn at normal rates by the most commonly used teaching procedures.

Although the visually impaired student with an additional learning problem might be placed in reading with a specialist in remedial reading or learning disabilities, the teacher of visually impaired students will likely have the responsibility of coordinating instruction in the basic communication skills. Regular educators have a tendency to contribute any additional problems which the child may have to the visual impairment, whether the additional problem is social, emotional or physical. Limited vision should play less of a role in the reading process once the student is provided the appropriate braille and large print materials and instruction in their use. After this provision, reading instruction should proceed as for normal learners taking into consideration special methods described in Chapters 2-5. However, such a smooth acquisition in reading is not the course of events for the many visually impaired readers with learning problems.

Although this chapter identifies visually impaired students with learning problems, these characteristics may also be attributed to normally sighted students with identified learning problems. Additional information is available in journals and books directly written for educators who work with sighted students who are learning disabled (Farnham-Diggory, 1978; Haring & Phillips, 1972; Ross, 1977). The term "learning disabled" is not used in this text because such a phrase is an official label analogous to "legally blind" and, as such, should be reserved for students who have been identified by the appropriate procedures. Nevertheless, the teaching techniques appropriate for children with learning problems should be of use to the vision specialist providing direct instruction in basic reading and writing skills.

THE DEFINITION OF LEARNING DISABILITIES

The formula for certifying students as "learning disabled" provided within the 1976 Federal Register is based on the concept of a discrepancy between measured academic achievement and expected achievement. This current federal definition also states that the "academic deficit cannot be the result of other causes such as emotional and personality factors, cultural deprivation, impaired sensory acuity, or educational deprivation" (Wilson, 1985, p. 45).

It is important to note that this definition does not automatically exclude visually impaired students from being eligible for certification as "learning disabled." An examination of the precise wording provides the clue to interpreting the definition. The term does not include children who have learning problems which are primarily the result of visual handicaps.

"The conceptual and operational definition of a learning disability has been one of the most debated topics in special education" (Wilson, 1985, p. 44). The difference in definitions bear more relation to funding for services and official recordkeeping than to teaching strategies which are directly applicable in the classroom. The visually impaired student with a discrepancy between expected reading and writing skills and current skill levels needs specific assessment and teaching techniques. Occasionally, teachers may find statements in a student's record in which a professional alludes to underlying problems with descriptive terms such as: inattentive, minimal brain damage, birth trauma, immature, or hyperactive. To the teacher who is frustrated with trying to teach a student new words when the student forgets them faster than they can be introduced, labels and definitions are moot issues unless they are accompanied by specific suggestions.

Labeling of visually impaired students as learning disabled is not the purpose of this chapter. The purpose is to identify the characteristics and common behaviors of any visually impaired child who has a learning pattern that is different from the majority of students of the same age. Once the child with learning differences has been identified, the teacher can select materials and teaching techniques to capitalize on learning strengths and to circumvent learning deficits.

CHARACTERISTIC LEARNING PROBLEMS

The particular characteristics of visually impaired students with learning problems may be as wide ranging as a 9-year-old's inability to remember letter sounds and letter names to a 16-year-old who cannot get to school with completed homework. The most common characteristics which the authors have observed in the majority of such students are listed below:

1. Academic achievement is below expected performance.
2. High distractibility interferes with learning.
3. Avoidance behaviors may develop.
4. Learning differences may be circumvented.
5. Learning in some academic areas may occur quickly.

Behavior problems also may occur in relation to learning problems, but they are rarely the primary cause of learning problems (Whelan, 1974). Gillingham says of her clinical work with the normally sighted, problem learner, "The child with specific reading and spelling disability, frustrated and frightened by his failure, may well become an emotional and behavioral problem. To attribute his spelling and reading difficulty to an emotional cause is to put the cart before the horse." (Gillingham & Stillman, 1960, p. 19).

The characteristic indicators of potential problems may be used to identify a student at risk of problems and avoid or lessen the experiences of failure. The student who was delayed in learning to read and/or write and later learned to read and write effectively still remembers the frustration of failure. "They have deeply ingrained in their unconscious minds that most devastating of all lessons — that failure can follow earnest effort." (Gillingham & Stillman, 1960, p. 21).

Academic Achievement Is Below Expected Performance

The visually impaired child with learning problems is typically not a child who would score within the lower percentiles of an intelligence test. In fact, the verbal intelligence scores for some problem learners may be well above average. Many visually impaired problem learners seem to have good reasoning skills and appear to be intelligent and ready to learn educational tasks, including reading and writing tasks. Yet, they show a discrepancy between their expected success and their level of reading and/or writing achievement.

Visually impaired students with learning problems may also have difficulty in mathematical computation and reasoning problems, as well as in one or more areas of communication. Students may have strengths in some facet of math or communications that will provide a learning channel to overcome other problem areas (Kirk, McCarthy, & Kirk, 1968). For example, a visually impaired student may be adept at math reasoning and may quickly grasp main ideas and make inferences in listening to a passage; however, the student may not remember sight words or recall details within a story. Once again the identifying characteristic of the student with a learning problem is a discrepancy in the student's skills in different types of learning tasks (Hallahan & Kauffman, 1976).

High Distractibility Interferes with Learning

The visually impaired student with learning problems typically is highly distractible which causes difficulty in controlling and maintaining attention to a task. Maintaining attention to reading or writing tasks includes being aware of important stimuli, blocking out extraneous stimuli, such as sounds in the room, and selectively attending to instructions from the teacher (Gibson, 1969). Sufficient attention span is needed in completing a series of steps to accomplish a task and following oral and written directions without changing the order or omitting a step (Strauss & Kephart, 1955). Remembering sequences of events and keeping up with materials also requires sufficient attention span (Mercer & Mercer, 1985).

Avoidance Behaviors May Develop

Avoidance behaviors are related to attention and concentration. The avoidance behavior patterns are typical of most students who are not having success in school. These behaviors are not peculiar to the visually impaired student who is not succeeding up to potential. Students may use several of these patterns in combination for coping with the various stressful tasks that are required of them in school. They are listed here because the vision teacher must have an especially "fine tuned" sense of when the student is not learning up to full potential because the learning activities are overwhelming. The vision teacher is the person who can help advise the regular teachers, the parents, and the student about what can realistically be expected of that visually impaired student. It is a responsibility of the teacher of visually impaired children to be sure that the student is actually able to complete the assigned class activity. Allowing the avoidance pattern to continue is counter productive. When the special teacher works with the visually impaired student for only a portion of the day or acts as a consultant to the regular teacher, the importance of not allowing the pattern to continue is increased. Guidelines in Chapter 5, Assessment of Communication Skills, can help the teacher of visually impaired children determine the student's reading accuracy, comprehension, and speed of print or braille reading. Guidelines in Appendices A, B, and C enumerate the grade level expectations in reading and writing that may be required of the student. A comparison of the student's skills with the performance levels that may be required may aid the teacher in planning and coordinating the student's instruction. Once the teacher has determined that the student can actually complete the task, the student may be convinced to put forth a maximum effort into completing the task. The following are a few of the avoidance or school "turn off" behavior patterns most common to visually impaired students. A much more exhaustive list can be found in books which are targeted for teachers of learning disabled students (Crosby & Liston, 1976; Hallahan & Kaufman, 1976).

An avoidance behavior pattern common with some visually impaired students who cannot achieve at expected levels is "passivity." Typically, these students may be considered "good students" when their behavior is the criterion rather than the level of their achievement. Passivity may be a personality characteristic of students blind from birth even when they are not under academic stress (Warren, 1984). Students who take this tactic are not being devious. They are only trying to be successful in the one area in which they can succeed — being "quiet." The student may work very slowly, failing to complete assignments or submitting assignments which are only partially completed. The student may even verbally agree to complete an assignment or to come to the teacher at another time for help; yet, this student does not turn in the work or come at the agreed upon time. Long-term patterns of passive behavior are easily established in children with very limited vision, and these patterns may be quite difficult to change as the student becomes older (Cutsforth, 1951).

A second avoidance behavior for many visually impaired students is to fill up the time assigned for a task with talk (Cholden, 1958). The talk may take the form of a conversation initiated by the visually impaired student with the teacher or other students. The conversation may be an interesting exchange or become argumentative, but the final result is that the academic task is not completed.

A third avoidance behavior is to blame the inability to do the task on the vision problem. Comments such as, "I can't see that," may be quite true, or it may be a rationale for the student's inability to accomplish the task. It is the vision teacher's responsibility to ensure that the media (large print, braille, audio) is appropriate for the visual needs (Spungin, 1977).

A fourth avoidance behavior is to blame physical discomfort such as a headache, or "tired," "hurting" eyes. If such comments result in the student being excused from the work rather than being provided with an alternate method to complete the work, then the complaint may be overused. The regular classroom teacher may take these complaints at face value, but the vision teacher can evaluate the underlying cause to determine if fatigue, frustration, or avoidance is the cause (Hathaway, 1959).

A fifth avoidance tactic that may be part of a student's approach to school is not really trying hard or going through the motions of the assignment without fully concentrating. Some students rush through a task and say they are finished. Others may work slowly without concentrating as they work. A typical comment for such a student is, "I don't know." Visually impaired students may exhibit other avoidance behaviors in addition to these examples in the preceding paragraphs. Additional behaviors may be identified in literature targeted for professionals working with normally sighted students with learning problems (White & Miller, 1983; Polloway, Patton, & Cohen, 1981).

Learning Differences May Be Circumvented

The specific learning deficits of some visually impaired students may be remediable, but the underlying problem may not be removed (Crosby & Liston, 1976). For example, the underlying problem of incomplete spatial organization which may have caused a visually impaired first grader to write reversed and inverted characters may later cause the same student problems with organizing the parts of a business letter, a task also requiring spatial organization. The student's spatial awareness may improve considerably, but there may still be a discrepancy in that student's delayed spatial organization and sophisticated skills the same student may have in other areas.

A sixth grade boy who had great difficulty learning to identify words until he received specific instruction in using consonant and vowel patterns to decode may use the same type of reasoning strategy to add words to his reading vocabulary. He still does not learn new words easily, but he can independently analyze the unfamiliar word for clues to the meaning of the word. He looks for the pronunciation of the word by decoding it into prefix, root word, and suffix. The potential problem is still present, but the student has learned circumventing strategies that work for him and, most important, he has the confidence that he can read if he utilizes different strategies. It is as one braille student said, "I can read most anything they put in braille if I just take time to figure it out."

Learning in Some Academic Areas May Occur Quickly

Once a visually impaired student is shown new strategies for handling a problem, learning may greatly improve in a deficit area. For example, a girl in a fourth grade placement who is virtually a non-reader may increase her reading scores on standardized material by more than one grade level with instruction matched to her learning style. The prospect for improved and eventually well-rounded academic achievement is quite good for such students (Fry, 1972).

Learning in some areas may not be very significant because of certain physiological and/or psychological deficits. For example, some children with cerebral palsy may never write legibly, or some poor spellers may never be proficient in spelling, or some children cannot seem to follow directions or retell stories in more than a three-stage sequence. However, these children may learn to compensate for these inabilities. For example, the child with cerebral palsy may learn to type as a substitute for poor handwriting skills. The child who is a poor speller can maintain a personal dictionary of misspelled words or learn to substitute a synonym. The literate child who has a problem following directions may help to overcome this problem by keeping careful notes of each step and carrying out the directions one step at a time (Mercer & Mercer, 1985).

Seven specific areas are identified below in which visually impaired students may have problems in learning. These areas are components of the mechanism by which new learning is acquired, stored, retrieved, and applied in new contexts. They are interrelated across curriculum from basic skills in reading and writing literacy to sophisticated thinking skills. When visually impaired students have problems learning in one of these areas, academic achievement may be delayed. For each of the seven areas, examples of learners with deficits in each are have been contrasted with examples of learners who have corresponding strengths:

1. Memory
2. Perception
3. Organization
4. Concrete thinking
5. Perseveration and fixation
6. Generalization
7. Language

In the following chapter, "Teaching Techniques for Visually Impaired Students with Learning Problems," these seven areas will be identified with specific recommendations for methods and materials to successfully teach students with problems in these areas.

Memory

The storage and retrieval of information in memory is an intricate neurological task that is not fully understood (Restak, 1984). Memory is interrelated to each of the other six areas of learning problems and is essential to any type of learning.

The process of remembering begins with the reception of information through the senses. Hearing, vision, and touch are the main senses used to get academic information. The quality of the information which is received by the senses is governed by the student's attention, perception, and the efficiency of the sensory processes (Gibson, 1969).

After reception, the information is stored. Levels of memory storage range from immediate recall with short-term memory to recalling information stored several years with long-term memory (Smith, 1978). It is the teacher's job to help students acquire reading and writing skills in long-term memory and to practice basic skills until they become automatic. Information which has been received and stored in long-term memory may be retrieved or remembered. The efficiency of remembering depends on the accuracy with which the information is received and coded into memory storage. If the information is received inaccurately or stored inefficiently, then the student will have trouble remembering.

The authors recognize that there are many aspects of memory that may be examined separately. Of the several aspects, two discrete mechanisms for storing information in memory have been observed to cause problems for some visually impaired students. The two important memory mechanisms are rote memory and logical memory.

Information which is learned in rote memory seems to be stored sequentially. Examples of information typically stored through rote memory are the lyrics and rhythms of songs, poems, spelling words, sight words, and definitions.

Logical memory seems to store information by association and classification. Examples of tasks requiring logical memory are identifying the main idea of a story, making an inference, integrating new information with previous learning, and drawing a conclusion.

Both aspects of memory storage — rote memory and logical memory — are essential for full development of oral and written communications. Students with learning problems may have deficits in rote memory, logical memory, or both areas. They may learn to use the stronger aspect of memory to compensate for these deficits.

The two vignettes that follow describe two visually impaired students. The first student, George, had strong logical memory and poor rote memory. The second student, Tommy, had strengths in rote memory and weaknesses in logical memory.

> George was an 8-year-old student with a deficit in rote memory and strength in logical memory. He was still not able to identify words in a primer level book typically mastered in the first grade at a 90% accuracy level by visually impaired students without learning problems. Since his visual impairment was cause by albinism, he was sensitive to high levels of brightness, especially glare, but he used his vision predictably and efficiently. He had great trouble with math facts and his memory for spelling words, either orally or written, seemed hopeless. When he listened to material, he missed specific details but was quick to grasp the main ideas, draw an inference, and identify an underlying moral. He could predict outcome and relate what he heard to a broad knowledge of current events backed up with a large and meaningful vocabulary.
>
> George had trouble sequencing events and any time-oriented tasks. His gross motor movements were generally uncoordinated. As he walked, his arms or legs did not swing across the midline of his body which is typical for an 8-year-old. His handwriting, which was laboured, resulted in neat, accurately formed letters, although he was not consistent in the motion sequence used to form the letters. He was more successful at other paper and pencil

tasks, such as drawing diagrams and geometric designs which were favorite pastimes.

In schoolwork, George was nervous about any interruption in the normal school day. He was quite inflexible, and completed activities in predictable routines. His organization of materials and working area was meticulous, and he jealously guarded his space and possessions.

In concepts of the world, George was knowledgeable but literal for his age. He tended to take a position and defend it without acknowledging another point of view. He had little interest in humor and viewed the interpretation of stories and events in a factual manner.

At times, George would fixate on a particular event and brood or worry about it so that concentration on other activities was excluded. Conversely, he could concentrate on something he enjoyed doing for hours.

George's pronunciation of words was incomplete and more typical of a preschool child than an 8-year-old. He had a large receptive vocabulary and at times could produce the precise word to convey his ideas, yet he spoke in incomplete sentences with little breath control or inflection. He spoke little in group activities and would have been classified as shy or even withdrawn around his peers. Most adults who talked to him for several minutes considered him intelligent and communicative.

George had a learning problem for each of the seven aspects outlined at the beginning of this section: memory, sequence, organization, concrete thinking, perseveration and fixation, generalization, and language. Because of these problems, he was not having success in reading. His most significant underlying problem was an inability to use rote memory effectively. His strongest underlying skill, logical memory, was used to compensate for the underdeveloped rote skills.

Visually impaired students, such as George, with strong reasoning skills but with poor rote memory may have great difficulty in learning to read successfully by the most commonly used methods of teaching reading. Sometimes these children are identified only when they have already experienced considerable amounts of failure. They may have attempted to use a few inappropriate reading strategies and lost hope in learning to read. The cause of the reading delay is frequently assumed to be their limited vision, and learning problems might not be even considered as a cause of failure. Consequently, a variety of teaching techniques and strategies may not have been tried. The extreme difficulty that these children have in learning to attach meaning to print or braille symbols that represent sounds and words might cause some teachers or evaluators to label these children "dyslexic." Since "dyslexia" is a term that has been defined differently by many different writers (Hargis, 1982), the term is inappropriate for use with students like George. It is a word that has been misused to apply to children with some reading delay rather than reserved for children with a genuine inability to attach meaning to symbols that represent words.

The subject of the second vignette, Tommy, was also a visually impaired boy who read print. Tommy had a strength in rote memory and deficits in logical memory.

Tommy, a 12-year-old sixth grade student, had been identified by medical documentation as cerebral palsied and visually limited due to cortical blindness resulting from a lack of oxygen at birth. Tommy's vision for moving around school was adequate, but he became disoriented in an unfamiliar environment. With academic tasks, his working distance was 6 to 10 inches from the page. He often tilted his head to orient what he was trying to see to a different portion of the eye, or to the other eye. Tommy could quickly and accurately read large-print materials. At times, he could even see very small print, such as that in a phone book or dictionary, but this better vision was infrequent. The occasions in which Tommy could see with unusual accuracy or unusually small detail were unpredictable. It was as if he could just "see better" on some days than others. Tommy's ability to see did not appear to be directly related to the external factors such as the amount of light, the intensity of the light, or the contrast. Nor could the efficiency of his vision be directly tied to a good or bad mood, the difficulty of the task, or to his overall feeling of confidence.

Tommy's academic strengths were word identification, vocabulary, English usage, and spelling. In fact, he was proud that he had found errors in spelling or punctuation in textbooks that had been overlooked by technical editors. His frequent comment when he found such an error was, "That is wrong. I never saw it written like that."

Tommy's academic weaknesses were in writing and mathematics. His writing was only barely legible when he used a pencil or pen. For that reason he had received typing instruction beginning in the fourth grade, but he was still a "hunt and peck" typist. The typing teacher's explanation of Tommy's lack of success in learning touch typing was that he could not remember the location of the individual typewriter keys. He also could not remember the correct finger for each key. Motor control difficulties also played a part in his limited typing ability.

Tommy had difficulty with most activities involving time, such as sequencing events or telling time. He was disorganized when using books and materials and was constantly losing items or forgetting to turn in completed work. He had a fascination with lights and sounds which interfered with his ability to concentrate. He would concentrate to the end of a page of work, but he had difficulty moving to the next page or to the next task.

Tommy had learning problems in most of the seven areas listed in the beginning of the chapter. These problems resulted in academic difficulties in math computation and certain aspects of reading comprehension, such as sequencing events, making inferences, and determining the author's purpose.

Students, such as Tommy with a strong rote memory ability and less efficient reasoning may acquire reading skills quickly and with little outright instruction. They may seem exceptionally "bright" during the first few years of school in comparison to their peers. Spelling may be especially easy for such learners. In fact, any rote memory work may be learned quickly and accurately (such as poems, songs, phone numbers, etc.). The child may even be especially adept at mimicking radio and television commercials or a favorite expression of a parent by imitating not only the series of words, but the inflection, cadence, and pitch as well (Fraiberg, 1977).

Reading comprehension may be less well-developed. Literal facts and one-step inferences may pose no problem, but understanding the main idea, drawing conclusions, and sequencing events may be especially difficult for the child whose learning strengths are in rote memory rather than in logical memory.

PERCEPTION

Children who have trouble with rote memory tasks are noted for having trouble in perception (Crosby & Liston, 1976). They usually have difficulty with decoding, spelling and aspects of writing. An essential component of storing and retrieving information in rote memory is storing the information in the correct sequence. Evidence of incorrectly stored sequential information can most clearly be seen in the analysis of student errors.

The errors that a student makes while reading are rarely random errors. Usually, there is a pattern of errors in memory or logic that prompts the student to choose a particular response even though the response may at first seem illogical to the teacher. By examining the child's errors, the teacher may be able to see the error in logic that resulted in the error in reading (see Figure 18). A student's errors may be consistent or erratic. If there is a consistent pattern of errors, then the teacher may explain to the student the pattern of errors and help the student learn to anticipate mistakes and hopefully avoid them.

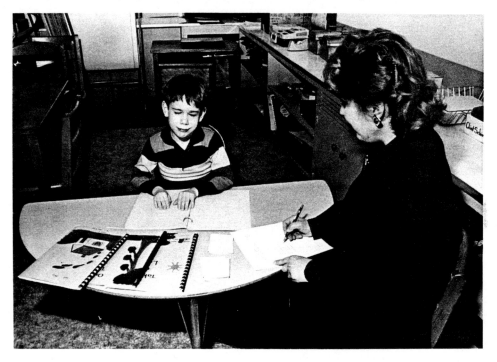

Figure 18. The teacher may observe a pattern of errors.

Errors in sequential perception which result in incorrect storage in memory may be grouped in six types: reversals, inversions, transpositions, omissions, substitutions, and insertions (Mercer & Mercer, 1985). Examples of typical errors in reading and writing will be provided in each of the six areas which illustrate how patterns of errors may be identified.

Braille or print students who have one sequencing problem, such as reversing letters, will typically have problems with other perceptual areas as well. Students will typically make multiple errors within a sentence or even a word. The more pervasive a child's sequencing problems, the more difficult it will be to find methods of circumventing them (Oreton, 1937).

Reversals

Some students who have learning problems that result in writing reversals, may produce letters written with a reverse horizontal orientation. Common left-right reversals in print are: "b" for "d," "p" for "g." For the braille student common reversals are: "e" for "i," "f" for "d," "ing" for "u" (see Figure 19).

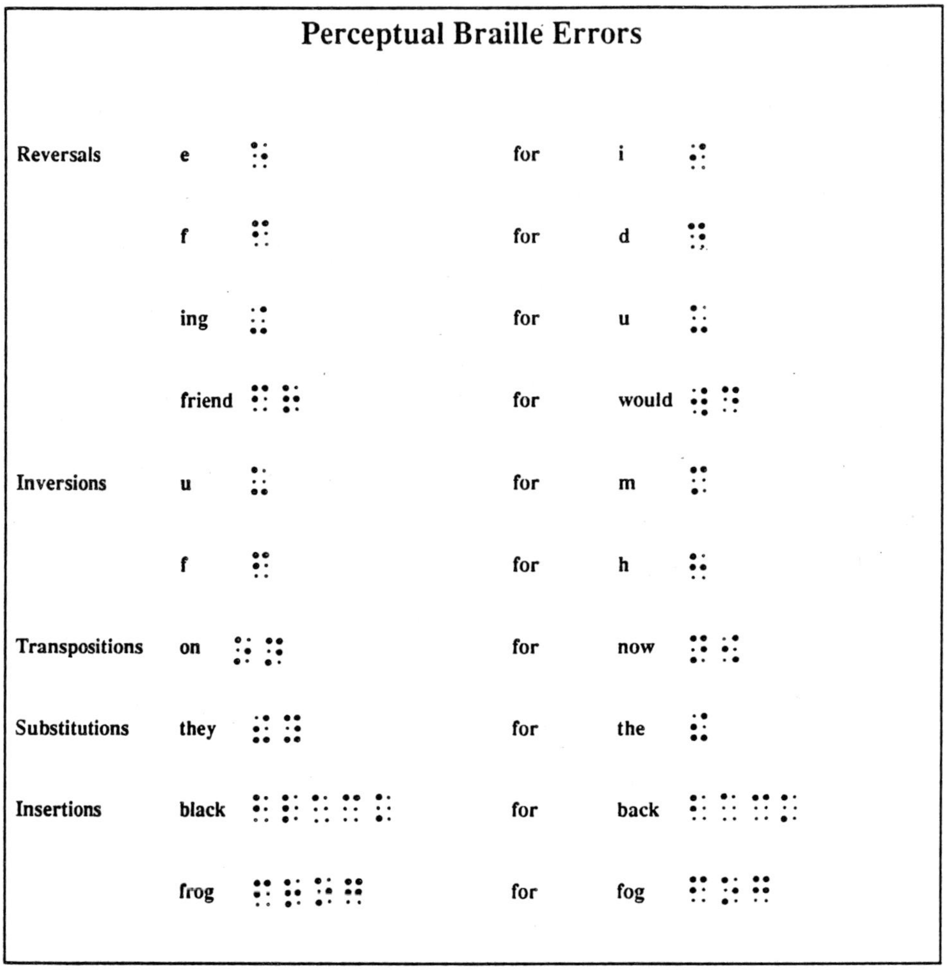

Figure 19. Perceptual errors in braille reading.

The reader may reverse the shapes of letters and the order of the letters within the word. One braille student read the word "friend" which is represented in braille by the letters "fr" as the word "would" which is written in braille by the letters "wd." In this example, each letter was reversed as well as the sequence of letters.

Students who read or write letters in a reversed form may also reverse words or concepts as they read or write. One such print student read the sentence, "Bob wants to *come*." as "Bob wants to *go*." The words are not similar in appearance but are alike in that both are active verbs. They are also opposites in meaning. During the same reading session, the student demonstrated other reversals by reading "dig" for "big" and "no" for "on."

Some reversal patterns in print are not so obvious. Another student's persistence in reading "me" for "you" puzzled the teacher until she discovered that the student did not discriminate between the letter shapes "m," "n," and "u." The same student frequently spelled words backwards so that "you" may have been perceived as "noy" or "moy." With the teacher's realization that "you" and "me" are both object pronouns and would fit the same predictable word order in the syntax of the sentence, the student's persistent error became more logical to the teacher. Once the teacher understood the clues the student was interpreting and misinterpreting in identifying the word, the student could be helped to anticipate the particular error and identify the word correctly. The teacher capitalized on the consistency of that student's particular confusion of "you" and "me" by informing the student of the error. The overall shapes and spelling patterns of the two words were contrasted on cards and in the book. The student was delighted with her ability to anticipate an error and avoid it. For the first few days she would share her success with the teacher by pointing at the troublesome word "you" in the story and glancing at the teacher for confirmation of her thinking. She would verbally prompt herself with, "I know one thing, it's not "me." There's no "m" in it."

Visually impaired students with a significant reversal problem may exchange the sequence of words as well as letter shapes and concepts. One such student read "Oh, Mike," said Jim, as "Oh, Jim," said Mike. Later in the class session the student read "dug" for "bug" and wrote "Tim" for "Jim."

Inversions

Letters may be written or read in a reverse vertical orientation. A few of these rotation reversals in print are "u" for "n," "w" for "m." In braille a typical inversion is "u" for "m," "f" for "h" as seen in Figure 19. Both reversals and inversions are more common in braille than in print because of the many more meaningful reversals and inversions. As with reversals and all other sequencing misperceptions, the significance is not in the specific errors but in a pattern of errors that includes reading and writing.

Concepts may also be expressed in inverse sequence. One student was reading a story about a cat that had climbed a tree and could not get down. He read the following sentence, "She wants to come *down*." as "She wants to come *up*."

Transpositions

The reordering of items within a sequence is a transposition. Common print errors are: "who" for "how," "stop" for "spot." A common braille error in which letters are reordered is reading "on" for "now" as Figure 19 illustrates. Such misperceptions involves the reordering of letters either at the receptive level of the memory or in the storage and retrieval of information.

Visually impaired students may attempt to identify a word by cueing to the middle or end of the word. Examples of disregarding the beginning of a word are the reading errors, "way" for "away" and "cake" for "make." In so doing they are reordering the order of letters in the word. They may pronounce those letters or syllables as beginning sounds. A student may be confusing the beginning and end of a word when the student reads "play" for "help."

Transposition errors in sequencing are particularly troublesome with numbers for braille and large print readers. Because the majority of large print and braille books will contain several volumes and are numbered according to the original print page numbers, visually impaired students have additional need for accuracy in reading and remembering page numbers. The carryover of transposition errors in sequence to math computation for such students is considerable, but math computation goes beyond the scope of this text.

Partially sighted students with a limited visual field may be especially prone to transposition errors. One 14-year-old student demonstrated a transposition type error in attempting to read the 20/80 line of a near vision test card that read 4376. The student read the numbers transposed as 4673. Such an error might suggest an error in acuity. The teacher determined that the error was in perception and not acuity by observing the student read the 20/80 line of another near vision test card that used pictures rather than numbers.

The same student demonstrated a tendency to make transposition errors in spelling as he orally spelled his middle name, Gerald, as g-a-r-e-l-d and wrote the name yet another way as "Glerad."

The following exchange between a substitute teacher asking a student about her remedial reading schedule shows transpositions or scramblings of a time sequence:

T: Tell me when you go for extra help to the resource teacher.

S: When I go in the evenings, there are two or three teachers in the room.

T: When is that?

S: When the bell rings for school to leave, then I go.

T: Is that after school?

S: No! (Obviously frustrated at Teacher's lack of understanding.) The bell rings at 12:30.

Omissions

Visually impaired students who have learning problems may omit letters in words or omit whole words in sentences as they read or write. The student may read the sentence, "The girl's dress was carefully washed and pressed." as "The girl dress was careful wash and passed." The writing errors of visually impaired students with sequential order deficits may show omitted letters and syllables from the written words similar to their omissions in reading. The most frequently omitted letters are the vowels (Gleason, 1984). Entire syllables may be omitted. The way these students misspell words will closely approximate the way they pronounce them. For example, a student may say and spell "enfirment" for "environment." Students may also omit endings when writing words and omit words and punctuation when writing sentences.

Substitutions

Visually impaired students with learning problems may substitute one word for another as they read, write, or speak. For example one fifth grade print student frequently substituted "the" and "they" in writing, resulting in sentences such as "*They* boys went to the track." The student usually could not see an error in the sentence even when prompted by the teacher. "They" and "the" are formed in the beginning by the same sequence of motor movements which may explain the persistence of the error for some students.

Visually impaired students with problems in sequencing may substitute letters as they read. In such cases, the child may substitute "list" for "lost," "mess" for "miss," and "slaps" for "sleeps." In assisting children with learning problems in substitution, it is important to determine whether they are visual (e.g., "mess" for "miss") or auditory (e.g., "cape" for "cake") or related by place or articulation. An examination of the student's ability to profit from prompts will help determine the type of substitution. If the problem is visual, an auditory prompt can be most helpful. The student's substitution errors in sequencing may become interrelated with under-developed decoding skills. Differentiating the two causes may not be necessary for students who respond to systematic instruction in using predictable vowel and consonant patterns to decode.

Insertions

Visually impaired students with sequential learning problems may insert additional letters as they read or write. Frequently, the inserted letter forms an initial or final blend in the error word. The most commonly inserted letters are "l" and "r" probably because they help form two of the three groups of blends (Gillingham & Stillman, 1960). The third group, the "s" blends, are all formed with the "s" in the initial position: "st," "sn," "sw," etc., while the "l" blends (fl, gl, pl, etc.) and "r" blends (br, dr, fr, etc.) are in the second position of the word. Common insertions of "l" or "r" produce errors in reading or writing such as: "grown" for "gown" and "black" for "back." Such insertions may be more common when the student is reading individual words rather than words in context. Frequently the error word is more familiar to the student than the actual word.

Some students who insert or substitute letters seem to blend letters from adjacent words. They may insert letters from words they have just read, such as reading the word "road" correctly and then reading the word "fog" as "frog" in which the "r" was inserted. Letters may be inserted at the ends of words, and frequently blends are again involved. One student read "set" correctly and then read "vet" as "vest."

The six types of perceptual errors in storing sequential information: reversals, inversions, transpositions, omissions, substitutions, and insertions are all types of errors in rote memory. These errors are most often seen in students who have difficulty storing information usually learned by rote.

Methods for helping visually impaired students cope with sequential error patterns will be discussed in Chapter 7. The teacher can help the student cope with such an error pattern only after carefully identifying the most consistent types of errors. A normally sighted student with one of the six sequential error patterns will typically have problems in all areas. The visually impaired students with learning problems do not differ from their normally sighted peers in this respect. Sequential errors of the type described are most common for students who do not have well-developed rote memory skills. They will have the best success with re-mediating their problems if they have a strong logical memory.

Moving back and forth within a sequence is another aspect of se-quential memory or rote memory. Some visually impaired students with learning problems may not have trouble in the above mentioned areas of reversals, substitutions, etc., but may have trouble in processing infor-mation that is out of sequence (Fraiberg, 1977). Such a student may quickly spell the new vocabulary words in a story and read the story in-dependently, but they may not be able to sequence three events from the story in order.

One student with time sequencing difficulties answered the question, "What was the best thing that you did this weekend?" with a litany of the entire sequence of events for the whole weekend. A conversation with the parent confirmed that the events were in the correct time sequence. This student became somewhat frustrated at being asked to mentally re-view events and then select one out of the sequence as the "best." The re-sponse was again the recitation of the order of events for the entire weekend, alternately and enthusiastically selecting and then rejecting each episode as "the best one."

Low vision print readers may have special problems with whole-word recognition if the children see words in fragments rather than as whole words. Several eye anomalies may cause visual information to be per-ceived in small units. First, a very restricted field of macular vision re-sulting from cataracts, glaucoma, retrolental fibroplasia, or retinitis pigmentosa may cause such a perception of words in fragments (Harley & Lawrence, 1984).

Second, the fragmentation of information may be caused by very rapid eye movements. These involuntary and jerky movements of the eye may actually become more pronounced as the beginning reader tries to concentrate on a letter or word. If the same low vision student has ad-ditional learning problems that make the task of reading more difficult, the processing of the fragmented information on the page will be com-pounded.

A third cause of fragmented vision may be in the interpretation of in-formation within the brain. Perceptual confusion within the brain may result in visual information that is fragmented. Whereas, the student with a limited field of vision or central field scotomas may learn to hold the book or paper at specific angles and distances for maximum vision, students with perceptual confusions cannot so predictably locate the section of the brain that will correctly interpret the visual information into words and sentences. For cortically blinded students, vision may fluctuate. The student may see a word or letter in one part of the day and several minutes or hours later may not be able to even correctly locate the page. The student may see very tiny images at one time and not recognize larger and more distinct images at others. The fluctuation in vision cannot be directly attributed to changing lighting, contrast, motivation, or other sensory information.

The child who has inconsistent vision may have visual behavior that one teacher compared to "seeing through a sieve." Another teacher described a student who seemed "to hunt for a crack in the fence through which she might get a peek." Some of these children seem to be at a loss to know where to look and how to hold the page or book. In scanning a page these children often forget the location of visual stimuli which may have been already identified. Their behavior is in sharp contrast to their visually limited peers who know where to quickly and efficiently position the eyes and the page to compensate for their very restricted field of vision.

> Bob was a braille reader with considerable sequencing problems that affected every area of reading. His medically documented, central nervous system dysfunction was quite uncommon, but his beginning braille reading experiences were typical of the experiences of other visually impaired students who have similar learning problems.
>
> Bob's syndrome resulted in difficulty in coordinating activities of the left and right sides of the brain. When he was 7 years old, his motor coordination was comparable to the developmental level of a child of age 2. His verbal intelligence scores were consistently over 125. The disparity between Bob's expected reading level, as indicated by his verbal intelligence scores and his anticipated braille reading level, as measured by motor development, was more than 5 years. Through a repetitive sequence of braille readiness activities, such as the manipulation of bead patterns, pegboards, lacing cards, and sorting trays, Bob learned to integrate and coordinate finger movements for specific tasks. His overall motor coordination and neurological development were still well below that expected for successful braille instruction. It was equally apparent that Bob's vocabulary and linguistic concepts were more than ready for reading. His potentials were disparate enough to suspect he might have problems in learning, and instruction was carefully planned and progress was monitored.
>
> From the beginning of reading instruction, Bob was encouraged to use both hands as he read. When he was not prompted, he read only with the left index finger. The right hand trailed along the desk top, to the chair, or his clothing. When the right hand was not paired with the left hand in reading, the information received by the idly exploring right hand would interrupt

Bob's attention from the reading task, and he would be unable to continue reading without help from the teachers. It was not so much that the right hand was of use in reading as it moved beside the left hand, but that it was "out of trouble."

The right hand did eventually become a functional part of the reading process by helping Bob stay on the reading line. Since Bob's spatial organization was under-developed, he had great difficulty in maintaining his place on the line as he read. He would frequently skip one or two lines above or below the reading line without being aware of what he had done. At times he would lose his place in approaching a new line and skip to the top or bottom of the page.

As he finished the righthand page in reading a story, he would often be confused about how to go to the next page. At times he might move his hands to the beginning of the lefthand page that he had already read. At other times he might turn the page back and begin reading on a previous page. Or he might turn several pages at a time. If the page was turned correctly, he might ignore the lefthand page and continue reading the righthand page rather than the lefthand side.

Bob's reading errors were characterized by multiple perceptual confusions. For example, he read the word "scream" first as "scram," and then as "scrash," and then as "scam." He would seem to add letters to the words on the page. The most commonly added letters were "l" and "r" to make a blend in the beginning of a word. For example, he read "slide" for "side" and "grain" for "gain."

As Bob was reading, he tended to carry over individual consonant letters and blends from previously read words to subsequent words. The blending over of letters into the pronunciation of the following words was most obvious when he was reading individual words. In the words with long vowel patterns such as "squeal," "pride," "slope," and "jeep," Bob read them as "squash," "plide," "plone," and "jep."

The introduction of vocabulary that followed a logical introduction of vowel and consonant patterns was essential for Bob. He was able to remember the braille configuration of new vocabulary words only with great repetition, but he could decode phonetically repetitious words by applying phonic rules. Bob was able to read on grade level after four years of individual instruction. His oral reading was still characterized by errors and self-corrections, but his comprehension was consistently near 90%. Bob is an unusual student in the degree of the disparity between his strong verbal skills and his undeveloped motor coordination. However, the types of problems that he encountered and the reading skills he did achieve are common to many visually impaired students.

ORGANIZATION

A general lack of organization is characteristic of the work habits of many visually impaired students with learning problems (Haring & Phillips, 1972). These students have persistent problems keeping up with everything from their books to their homework — that is, of course, if they remember to take their books with them to do their homework. The desks and notebooks of such students are typically disorganized. Even when the teacher intervenes by organizing the student's desk and explaining how to maintain the organization, the desk may soon be as cluttered as before. If the teacher sets up a system in the student's desk or locker for keeping up with notes, books, and homework the student may not be able to make use of the system. Older students may attempt to cope with lost books or papers by trying to carry all their materials with them in a satchel or backpack. One seventh grade girl carried a canvas tote to every class crammed with at least three braille volumes, a cassette player, and two notebooks until the doctor's warning of potential spinal damage prompted her to use the locker assigned to her.

CONCRETE THINKING

Some visually impaired students tend to be very literal and concrete in their thinking beyond the age that most normally seeing children have progressed to abstract thinking (Anderson & Fischer, 1986). As part of this concreteness they tend to be quite literal in interpreting what they hear and read (Cutsforth, 1951). Idioms and figures of speech may be interpreted in a rigidly literal manner (Lowenfeld, 1973).

One sixth grade student's answer to a comprehension question about a Greek myth illustrates this problem. The myth, Bacus and Philemon, was assigned in the literature book as reading homework. In the story, Bacus and Philemon are lovers who were rewarded by the gods by never being parted. In death they become an oak and a linden tree which are intertwined. The comprehension question was, "What did Bacus and Philemon become at their death?" The student's written response was, "They became dead people." The student's concrete and literal thinking could not support the imaginative thinking required to interpret the myth.

Another aspect of literal and concrete thinking is observed in students who understand one word for a concept or idea (Piaget, 1969). Synonyms and shades of meaning may not be understood. When classroom activities directly tackle vocabulary expansion through synonyms and figurative language, they may respond in frustration with, "Why doesn't the book just say what it means? Why does it have to go and use all those other words?"

Related to understanding only one word for each concept and idea is a second aspect of literal thinking—every word has one and only one meaning. These students assume that each word or phrase has one unique meaning (Duckworth, 1979). Multiple meaning of words and homonyms are confusing to such students. Their peers of the same age may no longer be struggling with the concept of multiple word meanings.

A common problem in concrete thinking is the inability to attach more than one meaning to a word, especially in the use of figurative language. For example, "The book says Joe's thumb hurts so badly that he could hardly stand it. Was his foot hurt, too? Then why couldn't he stand?"

One example of a student's inability to understand words was a totally blind student's fascination with the salad "bar" that was installed in the dining room for teachers and older students. To that child the only meaning for "bar" was of the disreputable establishment near his rural home, and the only connotation he could attach to "bar" was negative. He could not seem to resolve the conflict between the salad bar at school and what he had heard about "bars," even after he had explored the salad bar with the teacher and selected food from it.

Another teenage student combined the words "remember" and "memorize" when she said that she had to "rememorize" where she put her coat. To her, the concepts of remembering and memorizing were identical, and these words should have one word to express them.

PERSEVERATION AND FIXATION

Perseveration, the repeated initiation and continuation of one activity or the initiation of the same topic again and again, may be part of the behavior of visually impaired students with learning problems. The perseverative behavior may be bizarre and socially inappropriate. One first grade student was fascinated with plumbing pipes to the extent that he would crawl under the sink to touch them and carried a piece of pipe as a favorite toy. Another teenage boy repeatedly brought up the topic of Beethoven. He would continue to talk about his favorite composer even though the person to whom he was speaking was no longer listening. Such students do not pick up on subtle clues that the listener is not interested. Even when told bluntly to stop, they may continue on talking about the same topic. These students may have great difficulty carrying on any meaningful conversation because they cannot maintain their attention on a topic that someone else has selected long enough to communicate. They may have trouble in class because they are distracted from a discussion or because they are not listening and following directions even when the teacher gives individual directions to them.

Frequently, the perseverative fascinations are related to and triggered by loud noises such as police or ambulance sirens, a fire drill, or thunder. When the students hear the sound that is uniquely fascinating, all of their attention is focused on the topic for a considerable length of time. They may even repeatedly refer to the thunderstorm or tornado drill for days. Since their thoughts are so completely filled with one topic, other learning is limited or halted altogether.

Some perseverative activities or topics are often related to real or imagined fears (Cutsforth, 1951). Fears of drowning in the rain or falling in the snow, of being hit or captured by an evil villian, or of falling in a hole may be phobias for these students.

A related aspect of perseveration is inflexibility. Students who are perseverative may be quite resistant to change. Once such students have established a particular routine, they may be easily frustrated by changes that might seem minor to their classmates. For example, change in the daily schedule such a an assembly, usually a welcomed change to students, may produce an angry outburst instead from the student who is inflexible.

These students may be quickly frustrated when the change is related to classroom tasks. They may react with angry frustration to seemingly small changes in the classroom environment, such as: they must use a different pencil, the location of the paper supply has been moved, they are corrected by the teacher for a minor error, their books have been rearranged, or they are asked to take off their coats. The outbursts may range in intensity from continual grumbling under their breath, to self-abuse, or aggressive behavior at another student or the teacher.

Perseverative stereotypical behavior, sometimes called "blindisms," can disrupt acquisition of communication skills. All mannerisms are not distractive to a child while performing a skill in reading and writing. It is the withdrawal mannerism that takes the student's attention from the learning task. Stone (1964), in studying patterns of electroencephalagram (EEG) activity accompanying alerting and withdrawal mannerisms, found slow EEG patterns that are characteristic of drowsy states related to withdrawal mannerisms. The withdrawal mannerism could represent "the child's attempt to meet a stressful situation by creating a sequence of rhythms and intensive sensory stimulation that produce an altered and, specifically, a lower state of consciousness" (Warren, 1984, p. 30). If the teacher wants to gain the attention of the child and foster learning, something must be done to stop this kind of mannerism and bring the child out of a withdrawn state.

GENERALIZATION

The young child who is just beginning to read is uncertain about which distinctive feature is important in words (Gibson, 1969). For example, the words "Get" and "get" may look quite different because one is capitalized and one is not. The difference can be a problem whether the child is a braille or print reader. Two different letter shapes are involved for the print reader. For the braille reader, the shapes are the same but "Go" is preceded by dot 6 for capitalization. For some students it is best if the teacher doesn't frustrate the student by repeating that words beginning with upper case letters, "Help," and lower case letters, "help," have the same meaning. To the beginning reader, they may not look the same either in braille or print.

Punctuation that immediately precedes or follows a word alters the appearance of the word for many young braille or print readers to the extent that it looks like a different word. When capitalization and punctuation are involved, the appearance of the word may change even more significantly as in the following three examples: "Help," (-------), "Help!" (-------), "help." (-------) These are all common appearances of the single word "help." Experienced readers mentally classify these three appearances as one concept. To the beginning reader, the differences may be more noticeable than the similarities.

The lack of sophistication in thinking may be observed in the same student when the student has only one meaning for every word. The same underlying thought process is involved in realizing that "Go" and "go" are the same word and in understanding that a train is made up of railroad "cars" hooked together which are not the same as the "cars" in which the child has ridden.

Garry and Ascarelli (1960) noted the over generalization of the concepts of time and place by a congenitally blind student. As they worked on spatial orientation and topographical skills, they observed the child used both the words "here" and "now" to represent the concept of the current space that her body occupied.

LANGUAGE

One of the biggest obstacles facing many visually impaired students learning to read and write is their speech and language. Children whose speech and language have incomplete articulation, abbreviated and incomplete sentences, omitted or distorted syllables, or scrambled word order are at a real disadvantage when learning to read and write. With such language differences, children cannot match the sounds and sequences of the words they speak with words written in sentences. Since a major strategy for successful reading and writing is pairing written language with oral language, these students are at a distinct disadvantage (Gleason, 1984).

Some visually impaired students may have considerable problems with articulation (Mills, 1983). Such students retain the immature articulation patterns of early childhood long after their peers are pronouncing the majority of words clearly. The speech of some visually impaired students with learning problems is not only immature, it is actually distorted, in that one word may be substituted for another and many inflected endings are omitted from words.

In examining the research regarding speech and language errors of visually impaired children, Warren found, "The weight of the evidence seems to favor the conclusion that there is a greater incidence of sound production and quality problems among the blind (Warren, 1984, p. 198). The greater articulation problems in low vision students than in totally blind students may be due to the fact that they may be relying on their vision to imitate the lips and tongue movements to form words while the totally blind must rely on hearing alone. Mispronunciations that are barely noticable in conversation are glaring errors when they ocur in writing. A careful examination of a student's writing may show a close match to pronunciation. When looking at spelling errors, the teacher may discover patterns of misspelling that shed light, not only on the child's spelling inaccuracies, but on problems in reading as well.

Voiced or Unvoiced Consonant Pairs

Voiced or unvoiced consonant pairs are potential pronunciation errors (Mills, 1983). The reader can experience the effect of voiced and unvoiced consonants by placing the fingers on the throat and pronouncing two parts that differ in only one sound. As the reader pronounces "tan," notice that the vocal cords do not vibrate for the consonant sound /t/. Vibration only begins with the production of the short vowel sound of /a/ in the word "tan." If the word "Dan" is pronounced with the fingers in a similar position, it may be observed that the vocal cords begin to vibrate with the 'd' sound and continue throughout the word. Students who are confusing /bet/ and /bed/ are not differentiating between the unvoiced final "t" and the voiced final /d/ sound. The lack of differentiation is reflected in the spelling.

Another pair of voiced and unvoiced consonant sounds is represented by the letters "w" and "wh" at the beginning of a word. The sound represented by the letter "w" is a voiced sound while the sound represented by "wh" is unvoiced. Students who do not discriminate between the sounds 'w' and 'wh' may illustrate this by writing "wh" for "w" or "w" for "wh." Some examples of students' pronunciations that reflect the lack of discrimination are: "whanted" for "wanted," "wat" for "what," "whent" for "went," "wich" for "which."

Other paired voiced and unvoiced consonants are /p/ and /b/ /k/ and /g/, and f/v and m/n. A child may say "botatoes" for "potatoes" or "signess" for "sickness" when these consonant pairs are not completely differentiated. It is important that the teacher not introduce any of the mentioned pairs simultaneously to the beginning reader.

Long and Short Vowel Shifts

Students may not discriminate between long and short vowel sounds within words as they read or write. Common errors include lack of differentiating between words that differ only in the medial vowel sound: "field" and "filled,": "won't" and "want," "fill" and "feel." The confusion may incompass several words, for example, "sale," "cell," and "sell" may all be pronounced and spelled alike.

Phonetic Spelling

Even when students pronounce words clearly, they often misspell words by writing them as they sound. For example, students will often write "shure" for "sure," "Chrismas" for "Christmas," and "grate" for "great."

In an attempt to spell words correctly, students often overgeneralize an unusual spelling pattern. They may write "weighed" for "waited." Over interpretation of incompletely learned spelling rules are often observed when students begin to apply rules; students may make errors such as "shoeses" for "shoes," "helpped" for "help," and "choosed" for "chose."

As children attempt to spell words the way they say them, they frequently omit syllables (Fernald, 1943). Many children assume that words are no more than two to three syllables long. They do not attempt to read or write longer words. Some examples are "prizners" for "prisoners," and "probly" for "probably."

Syntax and Dialect

The example that follows illustrates the way that dialect may also interfere with reading and writing. A student was asked to compose a question and then form an answer over a passage read. The student wrote the following question and answer: "Name three things that the robot does." "He cleenup, go get the news papper, and takes out he trash." The question that the student wrote is in standard English and contains no spelling or punctuation errors. The answer contains at least seven errors of syntax or spelling. However, a literal rendition of the answer would sound very much like the student's oral response. Perhaps, the question has no errors because the student is modeling the question asked by the teacher.

Frequently, students will omit inflected endings on verbs as they speak or write. The following example of one student's writing illustrates how adding "ed" to form the past tense is frequently omitted. "Every person had bake or cook something." Conversely, students may overgeneralize word endings in writing and speaking. "They beed good." or "He goed to the store." are examples.

Scrambled Syntax

Some sentences that students produce with non-standard syntax are not reflective of their native dialect. In the following examples, the whole idea that the students meant to express is reordered: One student meant to say, "There were weeds in the garden, and that made it harder to push the mower." The student actually wrote, "There were weeds in her yard, and that made it harder for the mower to push." Students may have considerable difficulty expressing sentences in any other syntax than subject, active verb, and object because it is the syntax of the first sentences the child forms and the order of the words imitates the pattern of the action (Bruner, 1975).

Students with under-developed syntax will have great difficulty changing and using different syntactical patterns. Asking students to change a statement to a question is a task for late first and early second grade. Some visually impaired students will have great difficulty handling the concept at the fourth grade level.

Lisa, who was partially sighted, was considered "slow and quiet" by her first grade teacher. In second grade, when her verbal intelligence was officially measured at 110, she was considered "lazy." She was treated with a variety of enticements and reproaches for not "trying harder." Lisa felt guilt for failure to read, yet she did not remember words when she tried her best. The highest praise she heard or overheard was that her work was good, "for Lisa." Visual limitations, due to congenital cataracts, were compensated for by prescriptive lenses and large print books. Repeated testing by the speech therapist showed excellent hearing and no noticeable physical problem in articulation.

The speech therapist noted that Lisa confused certain speech sounds. In trying to echo words, she gave back "b" for "p" and "t" for "d" interchangeably and failed to reproduce several vowel sounds clearly enough to be recognized. Plurals and other /s/ sounds were almost completely absent from her speech. She used the words "a" and "an" interchangeably when speaking and produced such unlikely expressions as "a apple" and "an chair."

Lisa would often confuse the order of letters in words. She would look at the word "lamp" and accurately spell all the letters in the correct sequence, "l-a-m-p," but when asked to pronounce the word she might say "plam" or "malp." Sometimes she might spell the word "lamp" incorrectly as "m-a-l-p" after reading "lamp" as "malp."

Acquisition of new oral vocabulary through listening was slow for Lisa. She often mispronounced words that she had repeated clearly in practice, such as saying "ciilivized" for "civilized" in which the order of syllables is changed as the order of letters is changed in "malp" for "lamp." Syllables and consonants were frequently substituted as in saying "valoplate" for "evaporate."

Lisa's speech was not only incompletely articulated but contained words that she had never heard or would not be spoken by a child going through the normal mimicking patterns of developing an oral vocabulary and a grammar for the ordering and inflection of endings for that vocabulary. For example, she said "carely" meaning "careful" and "safeful" meaning "safe."

Lisa had great difficulty remembering names of people and objects. For example, when she retold the major plot of *Robinson Crusoe,* a book which she had listened to on tape, she called the book "Rosy Curs" and referred to the main character as "that man on the island" rather than by her version of the name. Her retelling of the story had many instances where she used the all purpose phrase, "the thing" for names of tools and animals. Friday, the island native who helped Crusoe, was identified as "The other man who helped him, you know, named like a day."

Lisa's reasoning skills were well-developed. She could make inferences and apply a rule, or understand the main idea of a passage read to her. Her logical grasp of cause and effect was evident in the joke she made to the remedial reading teacher as she was struggling with a story. She giggled as she said, "I wish those kids couldn't talk because then I wouldn't have to read this page." It was Lisa's strong skill in logical memory that helped her to apply phonetic principles and respond well to systematic remedial instruction.

SUMMARY

This chapter provides a summary of behavioral characteristics of visually impaired students with identified learning problems. The particular characteristics of visually impaired students with learning problems are wide ranging but in general academic achievement is below expected performance, high distractibility interferes with learning, avoidance behaviors may develop, learning differences may be circumvented, and learning in some academic areas may occur quickly. Seven specific areas were identified in which visually impaired students are likely to have problems in learning. These areas included memory, perception, organization, concrete thinking, perseveration and fixation, generalization, and language. Specific recommendations with suggested methods and materials for teaching were discussed in each of these areas in the following chapter.

CHAPTER 7

TEACHING TECHNIQUES FOR VISUALLY IMPAIRED STUDENTS WITH LEARNING PROBLEMS

CHAPTER 6, "Identifying Visually Impaired Students with Learning Problems," outlined the characteristics of students who were having difficulty acquiring basic reading and writing skills even with the provision of the adapted materials and techniques identified in Chapters 2-5. This chapter identifies some methods and materials that the vision specialist may try with such students without waiting for the help of additional support personnel such as a reading specialist, learning disabilities teacher, or psychologist.

The most effective teaching procedures for working with visually impaired learners who have additional learning problems are also effective teaching techniques for many other visually impaired learners. The purpose of these teaching procedures is to highlight the most efficient sequence of instruction for the best use of the learner's time. The sequence of instruction is targeted as the "must" learning—learning that is essential for basic reading and writing literacy.

Much of the material presented in this chapter was gleaned from books and journals designed for teachers of normally sighted children with learning disabilities (Gillingham & Stillman, 1960; Crosby & Liston, 1976; Deshler, 1978; Epstein, 1986; Fernald, 1943). The material is not exhaustive since there is much about learning disorders that could have been presented, but these illustrations are common problems noticed by teachers of visually impaired children, and the techniques have been proven successful for some of these children. Curriculum sequences which may be helpful are listed in the Appendices A-D already identified and in Appendix F, Objectives for Written Language, K-12.

In Chapter 6, seven areas of learning problems are identified that affect the storing and processing of information. These areas are:

1. Memory
2. Perception
3. Organization
4. Concrete Thinking
5. Perseveration and Fixation
6. Generalization
7. Language

Visually impaired students with learning problems may have experienced considerable frustration and failure before they receive the specific help that they need to succeed. To help visually impaired students with learning problems develop communications skills will require the close cooperation of the student and teacher. The teacher may have some success gaining the student's confidence and cooperation by verbally acknowledging that the student is having "problems" learning when taught by popular methods. For the student who has already been attempting to read or write with marginal success, the teacher is confirming what the student has experienced. By putting the student's frustrations into words, the teacher and student can examine the problem openly and attempt solutions. The teacher who is expressing the student's fears in words is using a very powerful intervention tool requiring careful consideration. The intervention is potent because the student's thoughts are special privacies. Expressing a child's thoughts in words should be reserved for times that the teacher needs the student's maximum attention.

The teacher can state the problem that the student is having in learning to read, such as "You seem frustrated that you can't seem to remember what your teacher thought you should know," or "You can understand things that are hard for other students, but they do not have your reading problems." The teacher may suggest that the teacher and student are a team that will work together to find a way for the student to learn.

As reading instruction begins, the teacher may have success with students who are mature enough to understand the reasons for some decisions the teacher makes about the way they are being taught. For example, if the students wonder how they can progress to more challenging and interesting books, they may be told that they must read 95% of the words on a passage and answer 80% of the comprehension questions to read outside of class (Spache, 1963). A guide for selecting recreational reading is a limit of one error in 20 words (Fry, 1972). The teacher knows that such a rule of thumb defines an independent accuracy level of 95%. These guidelines, which are basic to an Informal Reading Inventory, are simply enough for many students to understand (Fortell, 1985). They may not understand what a percent is or how to calculate a ratio, but they can understand that 90% is higher than 70% and that their reading accuracy is being evaluated in a specific manner. Students can become active participants in differentiating between the books that they can read independently, books they can read with the teacher's help, and ones that are still too difficult.

Enlisting the students' help in the learning process may be successful for some visually impaired learners who have not had success in reading. Others may have become so frustrated that they show no interest in any aspect of reading or writing, since such tasks have been adversive and resulted in unsuccessful experiences in the past. The students may view reading or writing activities as class time to be endured but not time in which they can allow themselves to invest any personal enthusiasm or interest. For these students the teacher may need to apply external motivation, such as posting each new vocabulary word to announce increasing reading success, or graphing the percentage of correctly read words, or praising "John's new reading skills," in front of another teacher or student.

MEMORY

As in Chapter 6, the authors have organized the discussion of memory into rote memory and logical memory. Other discussions of memory may use other categories (Smith, 1978; Gibson, 1969) to describe aspects of the storage and retrieval of information. However, rote memory and logical memory seem the best dichotomy for the methods and techniques that follow.

The most difficult part of the reading process for normally sighted students with learning problems is to remember individual words. Comprehension of the meaning of the passage poses little problem for such students once the words are identified. When enough words are recognized to establish some context, then many other unfamiliar words may be predicted from the context (Torgensen, 1986). Visually impaired students with learning problems have the same difficulty with word recognition. They may have difficulty recognizing whole words, letter strings such as a root word with a familiar suffix, or words identified by the letter-sound relationship or phonetics.

A considerable amount of rote memory, that is essential for whole-word recognition, is required for successful reading (Gates, 1931; Fry, 1972). The majority of words must ultimately be recognized quickly and accurately for reading success. Visually impaired students with learning problems are at a distinct disadvantage if they have trouble remembering the configurations and shapes of whole words. The majority of reading series introduce the most common words in the earliest books (Aulls, 1982). Writers in the area of reading use various terms to identify these words. Fry (1972) referred to them as "instant words," Dolch (1950) as "popper words," and Spache (1964) as "sight words." Hargis (1982) called the immediate understanding of these essential words "word recognition," and contrasted it with the process of decoding or analyzing a word not immediately recognized called "word identification."

One well-established listing of basic words is the Dolch Basic Sight Word List (1950) which continue to correspond to the high frequency word pool of the major basal series (Johnson, 1971). These words constitute over half of the total number of different words used in the most popular primary level basal readers (Mangieri & Kahn, 1977). A great number of these words are phonically irregular and cannot be decoded or analyzed by the generalizations of predictable sound-symbol relationships. For example, both the word "came" and "come" appear on the Dolch List of 220 most common words. "Came" may be decoded by the final "e" generalization, but "come" should have a long "o" sound by the same logic and should be pronounced as "comb." Other very common words have letter-sound associations that will be used in only one or two words introduced in the first grade level (-light, -ound, -ought).

Many words that are irregularly spelled and difficult to decode are introduced at a beginning reading level because even rudimentary sentences require their use. Visually impaired students with learning problems may have considerable difficulty remembering whole words. The student's reading accuracy may fluctuate from day to day. The words that may be taught most efficiently as whole words are nouns because they label a concrete object such as: dog, house, and tree (Hargis, 1982). These words seem to be easier for the student to remember, perhaps, because the student can match the configuration of the letters in braille or print with a mental image of the object gained auditorily, visually and/or tactually.

Verbs, adjectives, and adverbs require the association with a noun or pronoun to have the meaning. The following examples illustrate the association of verbs, adjectives, and adverbs for meaning: "Dogs *run.*" (verb), "The *big* car . . . " (adjective), "ran *quickly* . . . " (adverb). The most difficult words for students to recognize quickly are the words that fulfill a strictly syntactical function within a sentence. Such words are called function words by linguists (Dale, 1972). Words such as *it, where, these, so,* and *others,* which are used as propositions, conjunctions, and relative and indefinite pronouns, are least well-learned because they are less meaningful.

A teacher of the visually impaired should be alert to the variability of the repetition of new vocabulary words in the early levels of basal reading series. The total vocabulary load or number of different words used in a first grade basal reading series may vary from 250 to over 400 (Hargis, 1982). The total number of running words or pages may be approximately the same for the two series. The visually impaired student with rote memory problems may be able to master a small number of words if they are introduced at a slow rate and with much repetition. The number of times that a student must encounter a new word in the course of reading to immediately recognize its meaning without decoding has been recorded at 35 times for the student of normal intelligence (Gates, 1931). This level of accuracy that Gates defined is necessary for a pool of the most frequently used words. This repetition level appears to be less for more highly intelligent students with no additional learning problems and may need to be above 50 for problem learners. It has been calculated that "at least 30% of the words receive inadequate repetition" for slower, normally sighted students (Hargis, 1982, p. 4). Considering the challenge to acquiring reading skills, faced by visually impaired students who have fragmented visual images or misperceived tactual impressions, the number of exposures required to instantly recognize a new word might need to be even higher.

If the published reading series is using specific high repeat patterns, that pattern is usually referred to in the new vocabulary section of the book. Publishers may attempt to minimize the new vocabulary load by dividing the word list into "high frequency" words and words that are "unique to the story." The "unique words" designated by the publisher are still new words to the visually impaired student. As the student attempts to read the passage with many new words, the flow of the context that is so essential to reading the hard-to-remember function words is lost as the student stumbles over the unfamiliar words. The selection of a series with a high repeat pattern and vocabulary limited to the most common words is essential for the visually impaired student with a memory problem.

Providing material with a high repeat pattern for introducing new vocabulary will often require the teacher to prepare worksheets and cards for the student in order for the student to have enough repetition. To facilitate the learning of words that must be mastered as whole words, the teacher may write the word on cards. To give the student an additional clue to the word, the teacher may ask the student to use the word in a sentence and write the sentence below the word or on the back of the card. The sentence is more useful if it is written exactly as the student stated. The teacher may want to underline the word in the sentence for the print student. Italicizing the word for the braille student will be more confusing than helpful. Activities that may make use of the words on cards include:

- reading the words and the accompanying sentences to the teacher or another student;
- copying the word and/or the sentences;
- searching for all of the occurrences of a word on a particular page of the book;
- keeping the words in a box in the order in which they were learned or as the words accumulate they may be arranged by first letter.

To assist the visually impaired student with learning problems in recognizing regularly and irregularly spelled words, a variety of methods is necessary. Variety is important because repeating the same type of activity can become boring, and boredom and learning are mutually exclusive (See Figure 20). The teacher will need an assortment of activities to allow the visually impaired student with rote memory delays to learn a pool of whole words. The activities which are suggested are applicable for the braille and the print readers with some adaptations and are presented here to provide a springboard for the imagination of the vision teacher.

The card reader may be used for a variety of learning activities including pre-recorded comprehension questions over outside reading for older students. It is a very effective method for teaching braille dot numbers for letters and contractions for teachers who use that system of instruction.

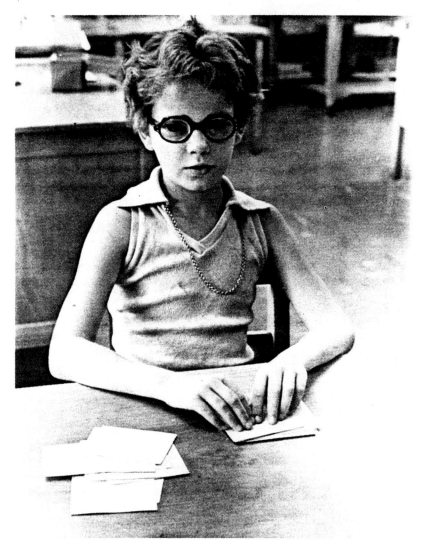

Figure 20. Many activities can be used to encourage quick and accurate recognition of sight words.

For the visually impaired student who is having significant trouble in remembering the shapes and configurations of letters, spelling of words, or days of the week, a different method of presentation may help. The use of rhythm and music can be very effective memory aids for lengthy or difficulty words. To help students remember the definition of the parts of speech, one teacher composed a song to the tune of Yankee Doodle which allowed the student to remember the definitions. The song began with the phrase, "A noun is a person, place, or thing, Like ball, book, and birthday . . . "

Matching

Matching can be an effective activity to teach word identification skills. The student may match copies of the same word. The words may be written on cards and may be exactly alike. To allow the braille student to organize the cards on the table or desk and relocate one without pushing others out of place, a sectioned tray or series of boxes are useful. A variation to the matching task is to have the student match the same word in various forms. The student may match a handwritten form as the teacher would write on a worksheet to a copy of the word as it appears in the reader, and the word as it is printed on the computer where the teacher writes experience stories or worksheets for the student. Use of a stopwatch or timer to monitor the student's speed in matching groups of cards may be very motivating. The times may be recorded and compared from day to day. The student is encouraged to use self-comparisons rather than comparisons with other students (Truan, 1978).

Same Or Different

Related to the task of matching is differentiating when two words are alike or different. It is easiest for the student with a visual impairment to recognize when two words are only slightly different when they are lined up vertically. For example, the words *help* and *here* may be the first words that the print student encounters that have the same first letter and are of the same general length and shape. These words also may syntactically fit the same word order in a sentence and so the student my incorrectly predict and make a reading error. Because of the similarities, the student must look at more than the first letters of the words to be sure of the word. When the words are written one above the other, the contrast is most evident to the print reader: help

here

Vertically aligning is not as helpful in braille and may be confusing to some students. Since unfamiliar braille words are read sequentially rather than in whole words, moving to a new line breaks the pattern of thought.

Labeling

Labeling common objects in the room is an important way to allow the large print and braille readers to encounter words in a meaningful environment. When positioning labels, the teacher needs to remember that the visual span of the large print reader may be beyond the arm's reach of the braille reader. Labels are encountered more easily if in predictable places, such as students' names on desks may be all on the top right corner or in the center at the bottom. The teacher should keep in mind that the braille label needs to be chest high if on wall, such as on bulletin boards, so that the reader can position the fingers to read. When the teacher is positioning labels on items, such as a box or basket for sorting or depositing work, the print label is most visible on the outside, and the braille label on the inside in an upside-down position so that student can reach inside the edge of the box and read efficiently.

Bingo

The teacher may use Bingo across many levels of difficulty. The task may range from identification of simple shapes to identifying parts of speech. Bingo has the advantage of having simple rules, and it is interesting to students at almost any age. To assist the braille student with markers that are not easily pushed from the space intended, the teacher may use push pins or tacks and some cushioning surfaces such as a cork square, a carpet scrap, or ceiling tile. Another method consists of placing the game card on a metal surface such as a cookie sheet or stovetop protector using small magnets as markers.

Categorizing

Sorting words that are written on cards into groups or categories is another type of activity. The teacher may vary the task and have the words sorted by matching vowel sounds or by sorting using beginning or final consonants. The student may even examine the same words on all three tasks using the opportunity to focus attention to different parts of the word on each task. Sectional trays or boxes speed up this sorting activity.

Cloze Technique

Using this method, the teacher selects and copies a reading passage and omits words in a particular pattern. For example, the teacher may copy a passage from the student's text omitting every tenth word. The student reads the passage and predicts the word that fits in the blank. The formula for omitted words may be changed and a new passage written for omitting more words or words of a particular type, such as all prepositions or nouns. The purpose of this activity is to focus the student's attention on the amount of information that is available in the words that precede and follow an unknown word. A problem with using the cloze technique with some passages is that there are too many different words used for the student to successfully predict. Helping the student differentiate "a," "an," and "the" may be especially effective with a modified cloze procedure.

The cloze activity is especially useful for the braille reader who must rely on the syntax of the sentence to identify configurations that are meaningful only by their position in the sentence. The activity may be varied by covering up words with small paper taped flaps and having the student predict words and later check for accuracy.

Additional materials and games for developing the rote memory of whole word, letter sounds, spelling patterns, and other communication skills are presented in Chapter 12, Instructional Materials and Games. The preceeding illustrative activities have been most effective for visually impaired students with learning problems.

Other Activities

The visually impaired student who has trouble remembering whole words through rote memory may build strong skills in analyzing the word by the component consonant and vowel patterns to identify the word. The process may be described as phonics, decoding, or linguistic, but the basic principle is the same. The student learns to apply the regularities between approximately 44 different sounds of English with the way these sounds are combined in words and written with the 26 letters of the alphabet (Fry, 1972). The use of decoding rules is necessary for the student to have a mechanism by which unfamiliar words are added to the vocabulary.

If the student has previously been taught by a sight word method, the student may be confused at being asked to analyze a word by individual letter sounds. The comments of one low vision second grader whose reading skills were being evaluated illustrate the student's confusion. He turned to the examiner with a quizzical and alert glance and said, "That's not one of the words I read." Such students may not be able to read more than 50% of the words previously read in a reading series, yet they will often recognize them as familiar word patterns or words they are "supposed to know."

Some authors and publishers have classified the teaching of phonetic generalizations as inefficient instruction because some rules are detailed and have exceptions (Gates, 1931). They argue that the time taken to remember the rules might be spent in learning individual words. It is true that some very useful rules may seem intricate and must be precisely correct to be helpful, but they may be the student's best or only hope to move beyond guessing and to begin predicting in reading (Gillingham & Stillman, 1960).

Using a little phonics among stories in a basal reader, may be less helpful than using no phonics at all. An integrated presentation of whole words and decoding are necessary for fluent reading in normally sighted students with learning delays (Vellutino & Scanlon, 1986). This integration is also helpful to visually impaired readers. The basal reader may introduce a pool of high frequency words and later may suggest procedures for breaking down the words into letter sounds. Children who can recognize the words as whole words have little need to break down the letters-sound relationship to read the word successfully. The activities in which the children learn the component letter sounds of familiar words may be helpful if the sounds of the letters are immediately applied to allow the children to read unfamiliar words. Simple analysis of familiar words may produce little carryover to the decoding of unfamiliar words but significant carryover into the spelling of these familiar words.

Many visually impaired students assimilate the generalization without much formal instruction. However, the visually impaired students with memory problems will need specific instruction in applying the phonic generalizations that are the most useful because they cannot accurately remember a large sight vocabulary and need to be able to decode to read.

The English language has evolved over centuries and new words from other languages are continually assimilated into the language so the language is not completely phonetic. The interaction of dialects and regional differences contributes to the complexity of the problem. The percentage of English words regularly spelled depends on the number of rules that are applied, and the estimates may range from 50% to 90% (Fry, 1972). When words of several syllables are included in the phonic analysis, English spelling becomes more stable, for example, the common Greek and Latin prefixes (inter, tion, sub, etc.) (Hanna, Hodges, & Hanna, 1971).

Sequences for the best order of introduction of consonant and vowel regularities have been suggested by several authors (Fry, 1972; Fries, 1963). The teacher of the visually impaired can use these and other sources for introducing the phonic principles. Some basal reading series will include an order of introduction of the consonant and vowel patterns in the teacher's materials. A few series such as the Merrill Linguistic Readers of the Lippincott Basic Reading are designed to emphasize the acquisition of phonetic skills first while introducing only the irregularly spelled words that must be learned as whole words and that are necessary for forming sentences. The teacher is encouraged to actively look for and compare sequencing of skills in word analysis. Several inventories and tests which contain subtests of such skill sequences may be a source of comparison. Basal series and remedial series may suggest alternative sequences.

Appendix C contains one list of skills by grade level for word identification for visually impaired students compiled by a committee of elementary teachers. Once the vision teacher has identified the student's current level of independent use of letter-sound generalization, then instruction can be targeted and subsequent generalizations may be learned and applied. The listed Word Identification Skills are those that would be observable in a student who is reading on grade level. In any one grade level, there will be students whose reading achievement is above or below the placement level. It is beyond the scope of this chapter to list the phonic generalizations, and the reader is referred to more detailed manuals for teaching remedial reading and Appendix C for Word Identification skills. Included here are specific suggestions for providing phonic instruction to visually impaired readers of print or braille.

Consonants are more quickly differentiated than vowels (Gleason, 1984). Individual consonants at the beginning of a word are the most obvious for the student to discriminate. The teacher needs to be thoroughly familiar with the regularities in spelling and articulation before beginning instruction. A few intricacies of consonant sounds illustrate the sound symbol match in English. The teacher may best impart information that the student can use when the teacher has a knowledge of both the common and obscure generalizations.

The teacher should avoid having the child produce isolated consonant sounds. Even voiced consonants produce little sound without the vowel, and unvoiced consonants produce no sound. Individual sounds should be blended mentally and the whole word pronounced. If the child cannot blend the whole word, then the teacher may help the student to blend the first letter or letters with the vowel sound, or the vowel sound with the last letter, and then the whole word.

There are three letters that do not represent distinct sounds in English. The letter "x" usually represents a /ks/ sound as in "box," and "q" which is always paired with "u" represents the /kw/ sound as in "queen." The third letter with no distinct sound is "c" which may represent a /k/ sound as in "car" when followed by vowels "a," "o," or "u," or represent an /s/ sound as in "city" when followed by vowels "e," "i," or "y."

The introduction of consonant sounds to visually impaired students in a readiness or first grade placement is most effective when the consonants are introduced first that have a sound that corresponds to the beginning sound of the name of the letter. For example, the sound made by the letter /k/ is the first sound of the name of the letter. However, the sound of the name for the letter "w" is /d/ not /w/. Students who are just beginning to identify words by using the beginning letter sounds will see the letter "w" at the first of the word and will attempt to make a /d/ sound.

The following consonant letters are ones that represent a sound that is the same as the first sound of the letter name, "k," "b," "t," "d," "v," "p," "z," "j." Consonant sounds that make a sound other than the beginning of the letter name are: "f," "g," "l," "m," "r," "s," "w," "y," "z." The teacher will have to be selective in choosing materials for introduction of consonant letters in the desired order. The majority of instructional manuals and teacher guides do not to use this suggested order of introduction. Frequently, the order is largely alphabetical or designed to match related materials by the same publisher.

Initial consonant blends or consonant clusters are two or three letters at the beginning of a word in which the individual sounds of each letter are articulated. Initial blends fall into three groups: "s" blends—"st," "sp," "sc," "sk," "sw," "sm," "sn," "str," "spr;" "r" blends—"pr," "tr," "gr," "br," "cr," "dr," "fr;" and "l" blends—"pl," "cl," "bl," "fl," "sl," "gl." Two blends that do not fit the above categories are "tw" and "dw." The print student's introduction to the use of consonant blends is comparable to that for normally sighted students. There is only one braille contraction in this group of consonant blends, "st."

Consonant diagraphs are consonant pairs which represent sounds different from those represented by the letters separately. The visually impaired student who is a "braille reader" will be introduced to single configurations for most diagraphs. The diagraphs are commonly grouped as /sh/, /ch/, /wh/, /th/.

The introduction of vowels to the visually impaired student with a memory problem is most efficient when the short vowels are introduced first. All of the vowels have at least two sounds that the student must eventually learn. But for the beginning learner who is already having trouble remembering, it is more practical to introduce the short vowel first because that is the sound the vowel will have the majority of the time in reading (Hanna, Hodges, & Hanna, 1971). Introducing each vowel sound with key words helps the student remember these sounds. Generalizing the vowel sounds to unfamiliar words is most efficient if the key words have the vowel sound in the middle of the word. The majority of short vowel sounds are between consonants. Some publishers suggest the use of key words in which the vowel begins the word (a = apple, e = elephant, i = igloo, o = octopus, u = umbrella), but the student will encounter few words in which a short vowel begins the word. Illustrating the short vowel with a beginning vowel may make the vowel easier to hear but words that begin with vowels are not typical of the words with short vowels. The student may help select the key words which illustrate the short vowels, but the teacher may guide the student to select words that are names of objects and that are spelled with a consonant-vowel-consonant pattern. To emphasize the sound of the vowel rather than the consonants, the teacher may select a set of words to introduce the short vowels that differ by as few consonants as possible. These illustrative words may or may not be the key memory words. Five possible words that differ only by the short vowel sound are: "bag," "beg," "big," "bog," and "bug."

PERCEPTION

Visually impaired students who are just beginning to read and who have problems with perception may have trouble with the mechanics of coordinating the movement of their eyes or fingers to correctly sequence the letters and words on the page. They may attempt to read the last word in a line first or try to spell a word by looking at the last letter first. Other students look at the middle of the word rather than at the beginning.

One technique to insure that students are looking and attending to the letters of a word in the correct left-to-right sequence is to have the student spell the word and point to the individual letters.

Sometimes children over-generalize in using rules such as those for adding prefixes or suffixes. For example, the child may add the suffix "ed" to "go" to form a past tense "goed." Usually the teacher can just repeat what the child said and the child recognizes the error. For some children, it is only after they make the error and are helped to recognize the error that they can really internalize the correct usage. Sometimes children over-generalize the meanings of words such as associating "stupid" and "stupendous" since they have the same first syllable. In such cases it may be helpful to look up the word in a dictionary to see the root words and their derivations. Another example of over-generalization is the student who read page number 113 and said "page eleventy three." In the example, the student was comparing a concept learned in reading 93 to 113. Another student who was studying short vowel sounds, read "want" as it would be pronounced with a short "a" vowel. The irregular spelled word is pronounced with an /al/ or long /ō/ sound dependent on regional dialect, but the spelling pattern led the child to generalize the consonant-vowel-consonant pattern for a short vowel sound. Gibson (1969) observed that over-generalization of rules is necessary for a student to learn the limits of the rule. The student is then ready to focus on the exceptions in light of the rule. Only with knowledge of the rule and some exceptions is the student really ready to apply a rule.

At the discovery level, fables and parables are useful to thinking more abstractly and applying a rule or a moral to a concrete situation with which the student may directly identify. Many of these stories are available in primer level materials.

It may help focus the low vision student's attention if the student points to the word. At first, the student's eye and hand coordination may be insufficient for the task. If so, the teacher may point with a finger or pencil. The teacher may even use a strategy in which the student's hand is held to demonstrate the correct procedure, directing the student's attention to the individual letters of the word. Pointing will provide a tactual feedback to the print student to help maintain attention to the task. Tracing the letters as the student says the letter's name helps some students remember the order of letters in a word.

For some students, the sequence of letters, or spelling pattern, is the most important clue to the identification of words. In fact for some print or braille students, the first two or three letters are named before any word is identified. It is as if they must verbalize the letter sequence for the majority of words to be able to correctly identify them. The following vignette describes one unusual student:

Shawn was a student with a very limited near visual field due to detached retinas and rapid involuntary eye movements. His field of vision for mobility was quite good, and he was able to skate and ride a bicycle in a confined area. As a fifth grader, his visual field and acuity were adequate to read small print. However, he had great difficulty learning to read. Various aids to improve his vision were tried. For a while in the first grade he had a pair of glasses with minus lenses that decreased the size of the print in the regular print preprimer so that more of the word could be viewed at a time. Teachers used a combination of a reading lamp with a reading stand to increase the illumination and place the page within the optimal range for viewing. However, Shawn preferred to lean over the desk to read avoiding the glasses and the reading stand.

From his earliest reading, Shawn spelled every word before he pronounced it orally. Even when he was able to read short passages independently, he continued to subvocally spell the first few letters of each word. When prompted that the spelling was slowing his reading speed, he said, "That's the only way I can be sure what the words are." Shawn had additional problems with handwriting. Written work was almost illegible, and Shawn could not read his own handwriting or manipulate the pencil and paper to make more than rudimentary corrections. The most difficult and frustrating task that Shawn had to complete was to read in a book and then write on a page. As in the case of other students in which both vision and coordination are quite limited, the accommodations necessary for the motor coordination posed the major teaching task. Shawn was provided with a portable typewriter and received typing instruction in fifth grade. He was a "hunt and peck" typist because he could not remember the position of the keys.

Of major assistance to Shawn was learning to diminish the erratic movement of his eyes through pulling his eyes tightly to the side or up. By holding his head so that his eye was in a position for eccentric viewing, he could read 8-point type. When he first discovered he had such control, he amazed the teacher and himself by reading the entire Weekly Reader in one setting, a task that had previously taken several settings with a magnifier. He had developed the maturity and multiple levels of concentration to minimize his eye movements and to maintain a particular body position to line up his body with the page. He could also block out external stimuli while fixating on the visual task. Even when Shawn reached sixth grade and was a proficient enough reader to score with a stanine of nine on the Stanford Achievement Test, he continued to spell the first few letters of the majority of words as he read.

Students with processing and perceptual problems often have nystagmus and/or visual field limitations. The official eye report available to the teacher may provide little information about the damage to the eye or brain as it affects the reading process. The vision teacher may be largely alone in trying various techniques for helping the student to use vision efficiently in reading print. .

Some students with pronounced nystagmic eye movement may be able to minimize the movement by pulling the eyes to the right or left corners. When the muscles that control the movement of the eyes are taut, the movement of the eye is often minimized. The involuntary vibration of the eye will usually continue to the same rhythm, but the actual motion of the eye itself may be less. Some students have discovered the method on their own and may be proficient in holding reading materials at a particular angle for the best acuity in the portion of the better eye. Others may have directed the eyes to one side to lessen the nystagmic movement for viewing specific objects for short periods, but they have not applied this eccentric viewing technique to reading. If a vision teacher is attempting to teach a student to tighten the eye muscles and lessen eye movement, it requires the consideration of several factors. Students need considerable self-control to be able to minimize movement of the eye muscles. They will also need motor coordination adequate to coordinate the holding of reading materials and turning the pages. Fatigue and the length of the reading passage are other considerations.

General rules are helpful to some children who, like Shawn may be having trouble remembering the sequence of letters for spelling words. These rules may be helpful in teaching proper sequencing in words that follow definite patterns. For example, in spelling "conceive," it may be helpful to remember the rule "i" before "e" except after "c" or when followed by "g." Such rules should be taught clearly with much written application only to students who need them and can understand how to use them properly. Rote learning of rules without practical written application of the rules with particular words has been found to be a little value. An excellent listing of reading and spelling generalizations may be found in Gillingham and Stillman's manual (1960). An abbreviated listing is in Appendix C.

Word cards may sometimes be used to assist students to see the order of letters in a word more accurately. These cards would contain pairs of words with the correct ordering and a similar word with an altered sequence of several of the letters in the word. Examples of such word pairs are "form, from," "spot, stop," and "flat, falt." The students may be asked to:

1. identify the correct spelling to fit a dictated sentence
2. copy the word that the teacher names
3. pronounce each word as the teacher points
4. make up a sentence with each word

These sequential steps can help the pupil to order the letters in problem words more easily. When the students are aware of the types of perceptual errors that they make, they may anticipate and avoid these errors.

Exaggeration in pronunciation is a frequently used method that will assist some students to sequence the letters in writing or spelling. For example, the teacher may intentionally mispronounce "separate" as "sē̵pa′ -rate" or "exactly" as "ex-act′ -ly" or "sardine" as "sar-<u>dine</u>." Accenting the problem syllable and using the long sound of the vowel may help the pupil remember to write the word correctly.

Another proven procedure in helping to sequence letters properly is to have the student spell the word aloud while writing the word. The student should check the word immediately after writing it by examining each letter in sequence and spelling the word aloud at the same time (Gillingham & Stillman, 1960). One boy who caught his mistake by checking a problem word said, "I know how to spell it, but my hands don't."

A third procedure that sometimes helps in the sequencing of letters is to spell by syllables. This procedure is especially helpful for unaccented medial syllables. However, spelling by syllables can be counter productive if the student omits syllables in the pronunciation of the word.

Suggestions for remediating a reversal problem begin with emphasizing left-to-right movements whenever possible. For the print students, activities may include underlining words as they appear in a left-to-right sequence, drawing arrows from left to right with troublesome words, and typing the words in large print with the computer to allow the students to see them being formed from left to right. The teacher may use the voice synthesizer to pronounce the letters so the students see and hear the letters at the same time.

Reversals, tranpositions, and inversions for braille are a much more difficult problem to remediate. There is a perfectly logical meaningful reversal for almost every braille symbol. (See the chapter on Building Word Identification Skills for a discussion of the intricacies of the braille code.)

Telling the braille students with persistent reversal problems specifically what they are doing wrong is an intervention that may prove helpful. It is more helpful to tell the students that they are reading an "f" as the letter "d" when it is at the beginning of a word. For example, some students may read "farm" as "darm." The students could be told that they are not confusing "d" for "f" in the middle or the end of a word. Such specific information is more helpful to the students than the general statement that they are confusing the letters "f" and "d." With specific error analysis the student may avoid mistakes more efficiently.

When a beginning large print reader has difficulty positioning the book at the angle for best vision, the student may often drop the book or lose the place. One solution is for the teacher to hold the book and turn the pages for the child, but this procedure means the teacher must be directly with the child during the reading process. The teacher's time may be too limited for such a procedure, and the student needs independent practice to build reading speed. One method to control the movement of the pages is to clip all the pages of each side of the book together. For small books, paper clips may do the trick. For thicker books, the teacher may use clothespins or rubber bands. When the pages are clipped the child is, in effect, handling only two pages. The student's attention can be applied more on locating the words and reading rather than manipulating the book. Clipping and unclipping to turn pages takes some time, but the student may spend less instructional time stopping to find a lost place.

Reading stands and easels, which hold the book and allow the low vision readers to sit erect and to tilt the book for best illumination, are invaluable reading aids. They are available from a variety of sources for tasks ranging from beginning reading to advanced word processing. The efficient use of reading stands is an instructional goal for many low vision students.

Some low vision students with delays in motor and neurological development may have difficulty coordinating the movements of head, stand, and eyes. Low vision students with learning problems may tend to pull the book very close to their centers of gravity (See Figure 21). It may be that moving the book toward the chest or waist brings it within better muscular control. Perhaps, the students are also blocking out external visual stimuli.

For some low vision students, it seems as if the student is dominating the book that is a potential source of frustration. The student may even kneel in the chair and lean over the desk. At times the student may completely encircle the book with head and arms. The student may steady the head by propping it on an arm or hand directly above the book. The teacher may find attempts to encourage the student to sit straight in a chair and use a reading stand to be ineffective if the student is not physically ready.

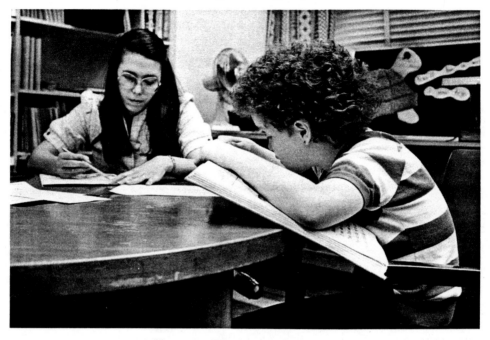

Figure 21. Dominating the book.

Some beginning print readers may not have the motor coordination for manipulating the many muscles involved in the eyes, neck, chest, hands, and shoulders to use a reading stand effectively. Permitting the readers to sit and hold the book as they choose, after providing instruction in several methods, may look logical to sighted adults, but the amount of concentration required for some children to use the stand may interfere with concentration on the reading task.

Helping the student focus attention on the correct word is a significant problem in braille as well as print. For the print reader, the teacher's problem is related to the movement of the eyes, the positioning of the book, and the perceptual processing in the brain. For the braille reader, the teacher's problem is not related as much to the movement of the hands as it is to the movement of the eyes of the print reader. The teacher can touch and to some extent control and prompt the movement and positioning of the braille student's fingers. But the perceptual processing within the brain is much more intricate for the braille student since there is a meaningful, left-right, top-bottom, and diagonal reversal for the majority of symbols.

For the children who are having trouble locating the place to read visually, it is suggested that a slotted card or typoscope be used to expose the appropriate words. This method may be effective for students with enough motor coordination and visual field to manipulate the card without getting lost or slanting the card at an angle across more than one line or print. For many visually impaired students, the manipulation of the card is just an additional task that adds to an already over-loaded memory. For many low vision students who track a line of print with head movements rather than eye movements, the coordination of the movement of the book is crucial. The use of a card to cover the remainder of the page or of a window to cover up all but the line to read is optimally effective when the teacher manipulates the card. The teacher may decide to invest teaching time in teaching the student to manipulate the card. For other students the time might be used to teach the students to coordinate the muscles holding their book. By the time the teacher has taught the efficient use of the card or window, many students will also have developed the coordination to direct their eyes without the aid of the card.

The special adaptations that are essential for some students may work against others. For example, large print may be essential for the child with congenital cataracts or glaucoma who has blurred vision or nystagmus which cannot be sufficiently controlled to read regular size print. However, large print could be very inappropriate for a child with a very limited visual field and good central vision. For that child, smaller than normal print might be desired to allow the maximum number of distinguishable letters in the viewing range.

A guideline in selecting print sizes is to ensure that the student can see the individual letters well enough to spell all the letters within a word when the words are in sentences. This procedure is a more complex task than reading the letters and numbers on a near vision test card or reading words in isolation. Recognition of the changing nature of type is important for the teacher of the visually impaired. Publishers of basal reading series use standard guidelines in formating and printing books. The majority of publishers use some of the following guidelines to printing across grade levels.

The type in a preprimer or other beginning book is larger than in the other books of the series. The type size may range from 14- to 18-point type. In addition to the enlarged type, many publishers add additional space between the letters of each word so that the individual letters are more distinct. They may also add additional space between the lines or skip lines. The type may be darker and/or bolder in the preprimer.

The type face may change from story to story, and the size and spacing may fluctuate as well. Changing type size and style is used by the regular publisher to add variety to the appearance of the book and to help the normally sighted student in generalizing the words learned in each story. However, the changing type faces may be confusing to the visually impaired print reader who must generalize a "g" and "q."

The large print preprimer is usually a photo-enlargement of the regular print preprimer. As such, it may be enlarged in the same ratio as other regular print books to achieve standard 18-point type. The resulting large type may be as large as 24-point type. With the additional spacing and the short sentences, the material may be read by a student who may not be able to read the standard 18-point large type in which the majority of large print books are written beyond a primary level. In fact, the visual task of reading large print in the middle elementary grades is more comparable to reading a regular print preprimer than a large print preprimer.

Sometimes students do not know how to turn a page correctly in a book (which way to turn) and locate the new position on the next page. They may turn pages backward. When the students get to the end of the page, the teacher may instruct them to "pinch" the corner of the page which they have just finished reading and then move it across their body (in the only direction it will move, left). If they keep holding the page until it is flat, then they may "let go" of the corner and move to the first word at the top of the page. Turning pages may be an additional problem for braille readers in that the early preprimers are only written on the right of the page. Braille students are conditioned to read only on one side of the page for beginning books and then must change the concept to read on both sides.

If students are having considerable difficulty remembering to begin at the top of the page and seem to be having persistent trouble in staying on the correct line in reading braille or large print, the teacher may need to help the students develop a series of verbal prompts that they can recite to remind themselves of what to do next. For example, an overheard comment of one visually impaired student was: "I'm at the end of the line." "Back up. Now come down to the next line. Now read."

Color coded prompts may also help the student's orientation. The teacher may use a symbolic color code such as a green dot on the top of the first word and a red dot under the last word. To cue page turning, a green line may be drawn down the right margin of the right page (indicating to turn the page) and a red line down the left margin of the left page (signaling not to turn backwards).

Students who are reading braille or large print may have overcome a tendency to be lost on a line at one difficulty level and may encounter the problem again when the format changes. For example, braille students may have particular problems when the braille format changes from double-spaced braille that has a blank line between each line of braille to single-spaced braille. The exact point at which this change occurs in a reading series is determined by the transcriber. The most likely stage is when the reading level indicated by the publisher is at a second grade level. The braille student may need worksheets in which practice is given in reading single-spaced braille for a few lines interspersed with double spacing to prepare for the transition.

Print and braille readers with spatial problems may become lost in reading when the format of the sentences advances from a new sentence on each line to continuous running text that wraps around the page. Some publishers have anticipated this problem and have gradually faded in longer sentences and continuous text in dialogue before using it in longer narratives. The teacher should evaluate the book to be sure that the change is not made too quickly for the visually impaired student to assimilate.

ORGANIZATION

Visually impaired students frequently have problems keeping up with materials. Books, classwork, and homework may be constantly lost. Time spent in searching for books and papers is time lost from instruction. Such wasted time is frustrating to the teacher and the student. It is one more indication to the visually impaired students with additional learning problems that they "Can't seem to get anything right."

The regular classroom teacher can help prevent much wasted time by carefully organizing the arrangement of instructional materials in the classroom and the requirements for the use of books and materials. The same general guidelines are appropriate for organizing a class to serve any visually impaired student since all students with limited vision need to learn to organize their environments. The teacher may not assume that if the classroom environment is organized, the order will carry over to the child. For visually impaired children with learning problems such incidental learning to organize rarely occurs. Organizational skills must be directly taught to these children. An efficient classroom will have the following characteristics: (1) a systematic location for materials that the student will need to use, (2) a consistent furniture arrangement that is free of clutter and obstacles to mobility, and (3) a quiet setting that is free of interruptions.

The visually impaired student must be helped to develop habits of systematically organizing materials. It is important that the student observe an efficient organizational system on which to model behavior. This systematic organization of the classroom is a form of structure in which the student can feel there is order and a reason for the rules that each is asked to follow to maintain the neat and efficiently functioning classroom. The student may begin to feel a partner in maintaining the order of the room.

A consistent schedule or daily routine is essential for the maximum use of instructional time. When the students are aware of what is about to happen next, they are more secure and better able to cooperate. The daily routine helps to provide the security of predictability and allows more time on the learning task. The students are freed from wondering about what may be required of them in the next activity, and they can concentrate more fully on the current class activity.

When the students are familiar with the class schedule, less time is required for directions in "housekeeping" details. For example, the primary student who hears the lunch bell quickly learns that the lunch bell is a signal to wash hands for lunch. The teacher with an efficient scheduling system may have established that students who are working on independent tasks may put away their materials and prepare for lunch without the teacher's direction, thereby, leaving the teacher free to continue to work with a student or group until the first group of students have finished washing their hands and there is room for a second group.

A predictable schedule is especially helpful for students with problems in sequencing. To help them remember the schedule, the order of the major activities may be listed on the wall in large print or braille. Some students may need the list near their desks or even on their desks. For children who are not readers, the daily activities may be reviewed orally. To help older students who may change classes every period and who have different activities every day in some classes, reviewing a weekly schedule can be a great help in remembering when assignments are due.

An example of a weeklong assignment sheet for a junior high English class is listed in Figure 22. Each Monday, students are given a new assignment sheet to be filled in with the specific "in class" and "homework" assignments for the week. It is essential that the assignment sheet be only one page long since multiple pages defeat the purpose of condensing the activities of the week into a manageable format. Moving on to the next page is equivalent to the changing of topics for many children with learning problems, and the second page would predictably be lost or ignored.

Week _____   Name _____

	Class	Homework
Monday -	English Grammer p. 46, comma review	Read "Ole Yellar," p. 146 Answer question, p. 151
Tuesday -	Turn in questions Quiz over "Ole Yellar"	Write draft 1 on topic "Once I was chased by . . . ."
Wednesday -	Turn in draft 1 Review "Ole Yellar" questions	English Grammar, p. 48, Commas
Thursday -	Turn in p. 48 Go over draft 1	Write draft 2
Friday -	Turn in draft 2 Quiz over commas	None

Figure 22. Weeklong assignment sheet.

The teacher can help to simplify the organization of the student's responsibilities by having homework assigned on a regular and consistent schedule. The teacher can also have the child check with the teacher at the end of each school day to summarize the assignments and homework and collect necessary materials. If one notebook is used for every class, the teacher can help the student use tabbed dividers to organize materials by classes. The notebook may also contain an assignment sheet, daily schedule, computer disks, etc. in such a fashion that materials are easily located. A more advanced student can often help motivate the immature student to organize a notebook so that it is more easily used as an aid to organization.

CONCRETE THINKING

As mentioned in Chapter 6, some children may need to develop more flexibility and less literality in communication skills. They seem to have a problem in learning that many words have multiple meanings or that different words may express the same meaning. Anderson and Fischer (1986) identified greater literality in congenitally blind children than normally sighted ones. In their comparison of the variety and flexibility of vocabulary of blind children, Anderson and Fischer related the immaturity of vocabulary concepts to egocentricity in the blind. Piaget (1969) observed this characteristic in normally sighted children. He identified three stages of a child's concept of object names. A child at the first and most concrete stage would think that the name of an object came from the object itself and, therefore, could not be changed. In the second stage the child may recognize that a name was identified for each object some time in the past but that the name is permanent. In the third stage the child understands that an object or concept may have several different names. A number of teaching techniques are available to help children move in to stage 3 of the concept of names.

If the child is having trouble understanding multiple meanings of words as "bar" in "salad bar," and the "bar" on the wall in gym, discuss with the child the multiple meanings of the word. Analyze the child's problem with the word "bar" showing the multiple meanings. Challenge the student to remember two different uses of one word. Focus attention on the desired word until the student is able to apply it in several different ways.

Another teaching technique for the child who fails to understand multiple meanings of words is to use vocabulary activities which focus on homonyms or words that sound the same but which have different spellings and meanings. Activities may be used to increase accurate use of homonyms. A game may be played whereby three different meaning clues are given for one word. For example, name this word:

1. It may be a source of water.
2. It may be a coil of wire.
3. It may be a season between March and June.

The teacher may emboss the clues in braille or write them in large print. If they are printed on cards, the answers may be on the backs of the cards. The child gets to keep all of the cards in which the key words are identified. The teacher or other student gets to keep the missed cards. The winner is the player who ends the game with the most cards. The same activity may be completed in a worksheet format with clues for several words on one page. A word pool of possible answers may be included on the page to aid the student.

The reversal of this task works well, too, to stimulate vocabulary growth and flexibility of thought. The teacher may assign words to stuents and have them think of more than one meaning or look up multiple meanings in a dictionary or glossary.

Another exercise to build the student's skill in correctly discriminating similar words is to emboss or print sentences on cards with blanks. Pairs of a key word are omitted in each sentence. The child is given a choice of words which differ only by a shift in accent to fill the blank. For example: "He tried to record the hit record last year" may be one sentence and the choices are: (re-cófd, ré-cord).

A third activity is to have pairs of word cards using various pairs of homonyms. The cards are randomly distributed to each student. The teacher may dictate a sentence using one homonym of the several pairs, and the student with the correct spelling may respond. For eample, different students may have the cards "hear" and "here." When the teacher reads the sentence: "I can *hear* the doorbell" the student who has "hear" may spell that form of the word and collect the card. If the student is incorrect, other students may challenge and win both cards.

Words that have the same pronunciation but three alternative spellings and meanings may be especially troublesome because three variable spellings are involved. Examples include: "their," "there," "they're;" "to," "too," "two;" "aisle," "I'll," "isle." The teacher may help the students focus on differences in spelling and meaning of the words with activities that have the students match the correct spelling in the sentence that illustrates the meaning. Such activities may be designed as games between the teacher and students, between groups of students, or the students may compete against their own previous best record. The students may copy sentences and do the matching as homework. It takes considerable time to prepare the cards but regular-size print cards can be purchased commercially from which the teacher can transcribe in braille or copy the sentences in large print. If the teacher develops original sentences, the sentences should be as short as possible and should be typical of the sentences the child would likely say or write.

Solving riddles can be a popular strategy in learning homonyms. The majority of riddles are humorous because of multiple uses of words (homonyms). The teacher can put homonyms on cards in braille with the riddle line on one side and the answer on the other side. Example: "Why did the silly Billy take a ladder to school?" Answer: "He wanted to go to high school." The student should be asked to find key words which make the riddle funny. Example: "Why is Cinderella never on any baseball team?" Answer: "Because she ran away from the ball." Riddles with homonyms can be placed regularly on the door or bulletin board for children to answer.

Idiomatic expressions such as "throwing his weight around" can also be studied to show the child multiple meanings of words. The teacher can collect these idoms from errors of her students or borrow them from print workbooks. The teacher can offer a prize to each child who brings an idiom to class. These collections of idioms can later be used for class games or individual exercises.

PERSEVERATION AND FIXATION

One way to control for perseverative or manneristic behavior is to keep auditory and visual stimuli at a low level so that the child is not distracted and tripped into perseverative behavior. If the teacher observes an external event that seems to trigger the perseverative behavior, that stimuli may be excluded from the classroom. For example, shiny metal, clicking heels, and bright bracelets may cause attention problems for some students with learning problems. Adjusting the shades to avoid glare and eliminating unnecessary noises as much as possible helps maintain student attention to the learning task. If the child is reluctant to make changes in routine wording, the teacher may explain in advance why the change is needed. The reason may be some external source which has a rationale which can be explained. For example, the students are not going to speech therapy when that teacher is absent, so they will be expected to participate with the rest of the students in a phonic bingo game. If the teacher can explain the reason for a change, the student may have more confidence in risking the change.

The teacher of visually impaired students needs to be especially aware of the role of the teacher in the learning environment. As is true for all students who are beginning to read, the teacher is the crucial element between the student and the learning that is to occur (Bond & Dykstra, 1967). The teacher is the most important factor in the learning environment. To be most effective, teachers must be aware of their changing roles in the dynamic interaction of learning. Since the voice of the teacher represents the teacher's presence for many visually impaired students, the teacher's voice may have a potent effect on the behavior of the students. The teacher, who can control speech volume and direct the sound to only one of the students in the room while being unintelligible and nondistracting to another student in the room, has a powerful tool. The teacher may change the volume, pitch, penetration, and emotion of the voice to prompt the behavior of visually impaired students in the same manner that the teacher of the normally sighted student uses eye contact. The "inquiring look" and "withering glance" for the normally sighted are analogous to the "silent pause" and "steel-toned voice" available to the teacher of visually limited students. The difference is that the communication cues are auditory rather than visual.

Teachers of visually impaired students may try to avoid common pitfalls of allowing too much sensory stimulation in the learning environment. One of these pitfalls is providing too much auditory stimulation through the teacher speaking too loudly. When the noise from a class activitiy is too loud, the natural human response is to counter the loud and noise with louder speech. This confrontation can become an escalating sprial of sound. The resourceful teacher will control the tendency to overpower the volume of noise with yet more volume and may use a low toned and well articulated voice that requires the student to stop talking to understand.

The teacher of visually impaired students should be aware of the possible distractions in clothing and fashion. Teaching low vision and blind students involves more physical contact with students of all ages for demonstration and instruction in reading, writing, typing, and other communication skills. Although bright colors may make the teacher more visible, they may provide visual stimulation for low vision students. For other students, the bright colors or geometric patterns may draw attention to the teacher and away from the learning task. Other aspects of dress and fashion that could distract from learning are long hair, rustling or swishing clothes, clanking bracelets, loose or hanging scarves, or necklaces. Perfume or other types of fragrances may be distracting. All of these aspects of dress and grooming are the perogative of the individual teacher. The teacher who is continually aware of the unique needs of individual students will maintain a professional appearance and avoid unnecessary distractions in dress.

For a child with behavior that needs to be brought under control, the teacher will want to use the least intrusive reinforcer possible to control the behavior. Verbal praise or a quick smile or touch are preferable to edible rewards. The vision teacher should be cautious in setting up a reward system to gain control of inappropriate behavior. The system of tokens, points, edibles, or time out may begin to be entrenched and become counter productive if continued too long. Such a formal system should be gradually phased out, and a long term system of variable social reinforcement should be initiated.

Another pitfall in directly using reinforcement to control behavior is in inappropriately matching the reinforcement in quantity or scheduling to the desired behavior. For example: One vision teacher was distributing edible reinforcers every 10 minutes for a student maintaining attention to a writing task. The teacher discovered that the student was distracted and off task for the first several minutes of the period and then the student attended to the task in the last minutes in preparation for the reward. She was able to change the situation so that the timing of the reward was not predictable.

As a rule of thumb, mannerisms are not easily extinguished, but the child may be conditioned by the classroom environment and the physical presence of the teacher to control such mannerisms. Some suggestions for modifying the behavior within the classroom are: (1) A quiet child may be used as a buffer for the perseverative child. The teacher may also seat the child in close proximity of the learning location. (2) The child may need a quiet work area. You can call it John's "office" or John's "work area." The area needs to be quiet, cool, and have adequate light. A dim light within the room with a bright light in the work area helps some partially sighted students screen out extraneous visual stimuli. The teacher may need to arrange a place where the child can escape and gain control of behavior and begin to think about the learning task at hand. The escape place should not be the same place as that used for punishment or isolation from the group.

The computer can also be used to help older children who are very distractible. The lighting on the monitor or speech synthesizer voice call attention to the computer. The immediate feedback of seeing or hearing words and letters helps to reinforce many children and keeps attention on the task.

GENERALIZATION

If a student is having trouble generalizing different forms of a word or letter, the teacher may say that the word is written in different ways. To help the student be aware of the several ways that the word is written, the teacher may prepare a card which has all of the forms of the word that the student will likely encounter. Once the student is told that the word may "look different," the student may be guided to locate the specific differences in "Oh!" and "oh." It is most useful if the child articulates the differences. If the child points to some part of the word or letter and the teacher talks for the child, the teacher cannot be sure that the child understands the meaning of what is said. By systematically teaching the distinctive features of letters, even partially viewed or blurred images may be recognized (Gibson, 1969).

One activity that can help the student gain speed in recognizing the forms of letters or words is to have the student search for that word or letter within a page. It may be helpful to keep the card that illustrated the different forms for reference so the student could check to be sure that the shape located in the book was indeed one of the different ways the word or letter appeared in print. To be sure that the exact match is involved, the teacher may photocopy the words from the student's materials and cut and paste the exact type style to cards. Different type faces may be contrasted with the handwritten form.

The braille reader does not have to contend with the different type faces of print. Braille students also do not have to learn a separate form for handwriting and printed letters, but the braille reader does have to contend with the confusing effect of punctuation and braille composition signs.

LANGUAGE

The child needs internal language that corresponds to the printed page for the best success in reading. A language difference may reflect family or regional dialect or it may be an aberrant pattern of articulation or syntax. Some researchers (Aulls, 1982) point out the dangers such as loss of self-esteem and loss of identification with family when attempting to change the child's dialectical articulation and grammar patterns. Other authors note that the more closely the child's dialect and grammar match the standard English in books, the more likely the child will be successful in reading and writing (Spache, 1976b).

The correction of oral language errors may be done individually and at the moment the child actually uses the incorrect pronunciation. Drills will not be as effective as the real life spoken or written language of the child. One technique of teaching correct usage is to repeat exactly what the children have said without corrections to see if they recognize it as something the teacher would not say.

The teacher may concentrate on the mispronunciations which are easiest to change; for example, the "m's" and "p's" formed near the front of the mouth have the most obvious exterior lip movements. Children with vision can see the movements. Blind children can feel the difference in movements and the accompanying air movements. The child who is saying "wif" instead of "with" can place a hand in front of the mouth and the teacher's mouth to feel the difference. The "f" makes an upward movement of air and the "th" makes a downward air movement.

A strong phonetic program in the early grades can help the child with an articulation problem focus on different sounds of consonants and vowels in words and the patterns of sound symbol relationships in the English language. By learning how to articulate correctly in reading, the child leans to carry this skill over to speaking (Gillingham & Stillman, 1960).

Some students do not differentiate between several words (barn, burn, bark, born) using one common sound for all of these words. Perhaps, they do not clearly understand the different meanings as well. The teacher may help contrast the differences in spellings by aligning the words vertically on a card for print students. The teacher can also help by distinctly pronouncing one word and having the student point to the written word simultaneously. The teacher can have the child read with an exaggerated inflection going back and forth between problem words until the distinctions are learned. To emphasize the meaning differences in words with similar sounds, the child can use the words in sentences orally, later copying the sentences. If a student confuses or swaps similar words in reading, the student may have an even greater problem in writing these words. Thus, the instructional time spent in reading to differentiate closely phonetic yet distinctly different words may help avoid spelling problems. Indeed, a case may be made that some students first realize the different pronunciation of similar sounding words by observing the differences in spelling.

Targeting instruction specifically on grammar for upper elementary and junior high students may help these students to express themselves more correctly both orally and in writing. One method used with these children is to individually correct the students just after the mistake is made. This correction may be embarrassing to the students if done too frequently, and it may become part of their self-image to use poor grammar.

The teacher may want to make a list of the students' grammatical errors that they make in writing. The teacher may write out worksheets with typical errors and have students find the errors. One teacher collected a notebook of double negatives that her children had generated in a daily share time. She transcribed them into print and braille and used them in group activities and games. These games were devised to find errors and to restate sentences correctly.

Another high school teacher kept a jar on her desk so that children who made grammatical errors could donate loose change. If a student made an error, another student might identify the error and state the sentence correctly. When the pot of change reached a certain amount, the class had a party. The teacher can also be one of the group in this game.

Some oral and written errors in grammar are less related to dialect than underdeveloped language syntax. The student who omits essential words in writing or endings from words, may be simply careless, or may actually speak with such abbreviated grammar. Some students exchange one word for another ("they" for "the") in writing. The written sentences produced do not sound like fluent language when read aloud. The teacher should avoid saying "look and tell me what is wrong" because the children will usually read what they intended to write. Alerting the student to the specific error of swapping "they" for "the" helps some students anticipate and avoid errors. Targeting only one error at a time is the most effective remedial method. If a word is written incorrectly, the teacher may help the student erase the whole word and write it correctly from the beginning. Erasing the entire word and rewriting from the beginning rather than erasing and repeating portions of an error in a word seems important for some visually impaired students. The teacher may help the child to build a pattern in connecting the motor and language components of the word. Once the word is written correctly in a sentence, the child may compare it to the models of the correct use of the troublesome words. When the student finds an error and verbalizes how the two words are different, a major step in anticipating future errors has been made.

The following books and supplementary materials are available in braille and large print. They may be helpful to students who are having problems in understanding multiple meanings and general vocabulary development.

The Specific Skills Series contains one strand called Working with Sound. This strand has phonics study at the primary level ("A" to "C") and vocabulary study in the most advanced levels which go from levels "D" to "L." Level "F" begins an intense study of Latin and Greek prefixes and suffixes. By studying prefixes, suffixes, and root words, students can systematically build additional vocabulary. A similar series is the D&W Supportive Reading Skills. This series also follows a systematic and sequential study of words (See Figure 23).

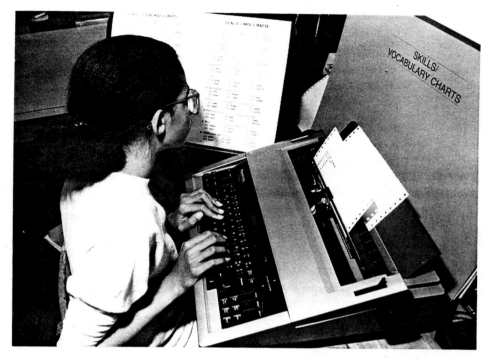

Figure 23. Supplemental materials provide a systematic word study.

The L&L Multiple Skill Series is designed as a vocabulary builder by using word studies as a part of the total reading process. Levels are available for second through ninth grade. The vocabulary of visually impaired students needs additional constant attention (Anderson & Fischer, 1986). Some children may be severely penalized in reading because of failure to develop reading and listening vocabularies. The SRA Reading Laboratory contains short reading passages in which building vocabulary is a goal of the activities (small print only). This series is only available in regular print.

The Reader's Digest Reading Skill Builders is available in large print and braille. It provides vocabulary introduction and drill within short stories. These materials are especially useful with older students because the content is mature. Reading levels range from first through ninth grades.

SUMMARY

The previous chapter, Identifying Visually Impaired Students With Learning Problems, describes typical behaviors in the areas of: memory, perception, organization, concrete thinking, perseveration and fixation, generalization, and language. This chapter has described specific teaching strategies and materials that can assist the vision specialist in providing instruction to students whose achievements are below expectations.

The student who will profit the most from the instructional strategies suggested in this chapter is the one who can apply and generalize rules for spelling, writing, and the other communication skills. A sampling of the scope of materials and techniques that have proven effective for visually impaired children with learning problems has been presented. For additional ideas, the vision specialist may refer to the references cited. The teacher's best resource for ideas comes from individual creativity and cooperation with the child in a partnership for learning.

CHAPTER 8

DEVELOPING WRITING SKILLS

WRITTEN EXPRESSION for visually impaired children is a natural outgrowth of their oral expression. Visually impaired children who are beginning to write have learned that reading a story is similar to listening to a recorded story. The next natural step is for the children to write (or record) themselves. Children with normal or partial vision may first experience writing by observing adults writing notes or letters. For the children who will use braille, the first observation of writing in their medium may be as the teacher embosses dots with the braille writer.

Writing skills include developing the mechanics of writing and learning to express ideas. Developing skills in expressing ideas through the medium of writing is a natural part of the language arts curriculum for all students and is not unique to visually impaired students. Appendix F, Objectives for Written Language, K-12, provides an overview of the continuum of written language skills. The mechanics of writing include the operation of the writing tools as the students apply the use of skills in spelling, spacing, punctuation, and grammar to express ideas. This chapter discusses aspects of writing that are unique to visually impaired learners. Sections include handwriting for low vision students, signature writing for blind students, braille writing, and typing skills.

HANDWRITING FOR LOW VISION STUDENTS

Just as reading is used in most school subjects, handwriting is also an essential communication tool. The low vision child who is a print reader must rely at times on handwriting skills to communicate through class notes, assignments, and tests. Typing and word processing are also important tools which can be used to supplement handwriting. Handwriting is a complex skill dependent on the integration of many skills, such as fine motor coordination, spelling, sentence construction, and using rules of grammar. All are necessary to communicate ideas through writing.

Ordinarily, techniques for teaching handwriting to visually impaired children are very similar to the techniques used with normally sighted children. The teacher who is preparing to teach manuscript or cursive handwriting to visually impaired students should be thoroughly familiar with the handwriting instruction sequence suggested by publishers of materials for normally sighted students. The suggested motor sequences for the letters are quite consistent across publishers so that a wide variety of comparable handwriting materials are available. Practicing standard handwriting on specific writing activities and applying standard handwriting to other classwork will foster neat, legible manuscript and cursive writing for many visually impaired students. Adaptations of standard handwriting techniques for use with visually impaired students have included using pencils or markers with bolder and darker strokes, experimenting with various colored lines for contrast, using wider and/ or raised line paper, and using paper with a dull finish. However, some low vision children have special handwriting difficulties and most blind children have difficulty in learning to sign their names. Handwriting techniques will be discussed in this chapter for both low vision and blind individuals.

Familiarity with typical handwriting errors may be helpful in teaching normally sighted students with writing problems. With a familiarity of the typical types of writing problems that many students may encounter, teachers may help students anticipate and avoid such errors. The writing errors of low vision students are similar to those of normally sighted students and additional types of errors may occur as well. Figure 1 illustrates samples of common writing errors of low vision students. Low vision students' common writing errors are illustrated in cursive and manuscript, because the majority of these writing errors are common to both. With a knowledge of such error patterns, the teachers of visually impaired children are better able to select and adapt standard print materials to minimize such errors in their students' writing.

The student may space letters unevenly within words. Some letters may be (1) far apart, and others (2) almost on top of each other. Letters within words may be evenly spaced, but words may (3) run together resulting in one giant "word" on each writing line. The orientation of letters and words between the writing lines may follow in one of two patterns. One student may appear to (4) ignore the lines on the page altogether and produce letters that either are suspended above the line or fall on or below the line seemingly at random. Another student may be (5) scupulously conscious of the lines of the page and avoid writing on them at any time. Thus, the letters that should extend below the writing line are crowded together above the line.

The formation of individual letters may be very inconsistent. The precise sequence of motor movements involved in forming letters may not become automatic with practice. It is as if the student is "copying" either a mental image of the shapes of letters or the model provided by the teacher. For example, (6) the manuscript letter "b" may be made in several different sequences of strokes, even within the same words. In the manuscript writing sample in Figure 24, the first "b" in the word "baby" was made by two separate strokes of the pencil and consisted of a straight line starting from the bottom upward and followed by a clockwise circle. The second "b," although looking in final form much like the first, was made by one stroke of the pencil starting from the top of the letter and moving downward, ending in a counter clockwise loop or circle.

Students who are using cursive writing may also use different motor sequences (see line 6, Figure 24). For example, the first letter "a" in the word "alarm" was written by a full clockwise circle and the second "a" by a full counter clockwise circle. Neither of these motor sequences are the half-circle and reverse to a counter clockwise method suggested by most handwriting instructional materials (Zaner & Blozer, 1974).

The letters students write may (7) slant in various directions and may change within a single word. (8) The size of the letters may also vary within the same word. For letters that have the same shape for capital and lower case but differ in size, many students write the same size letter for both capital and lower case form; or the students may change the size of the same letter within a word. Parts of (9) letters and (10) words may be omitted in writing. Experience shows that most common omissions are the inflected endings of words which make them fit syntactically into a standard English sentence (ed, -ing, 's). Also omitted are suffixes, punctuation, and capitalization.

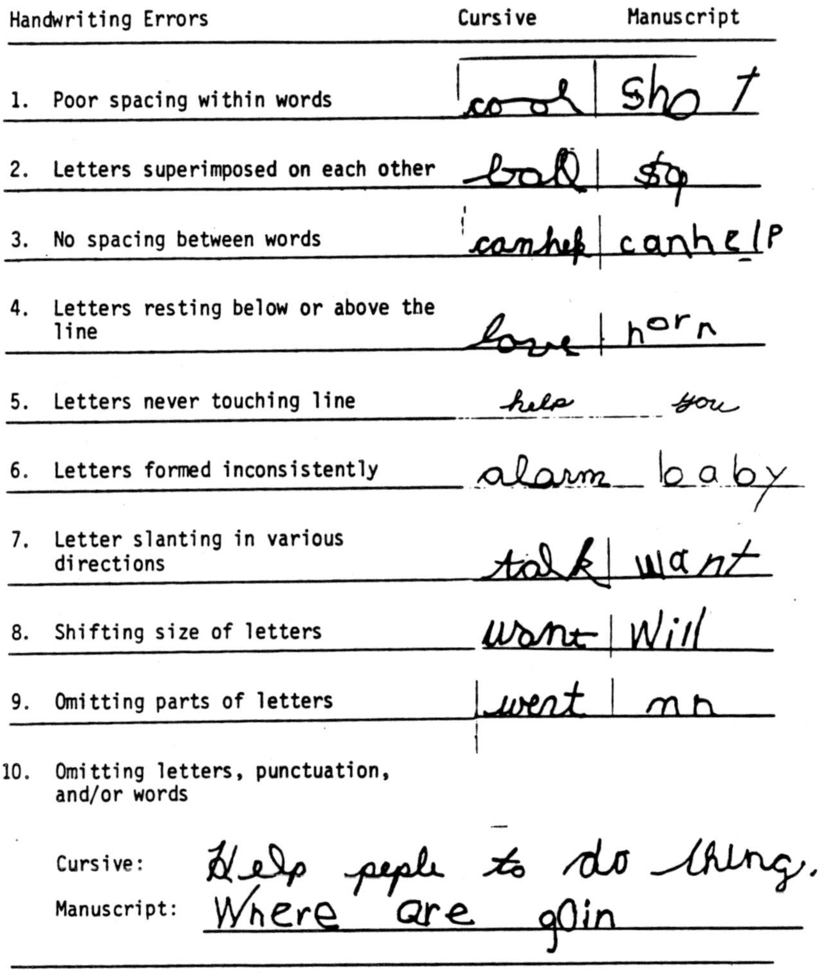

Handwriting Errors	Cursive	Manuscript
1. Poor spacing within words	*cool*	*sho t*
2. Letters superimposed on each other	*ball*	*sto*
3. No spacing between words	*canhelp*	*canhelP*
4. Letters resting below or above the line	*love*	*horn*
5. Letters never touching line	*help*	*you*
6. Letters formed inconsistently	*alarm*	*baby*
7. Letter slanting in various directions	*talk*	*want*
8. Shifting size of letters	*wont*	*Will*
9. Omitting parts of letters	*went*	*nn*
10. Omitting letters, punctuation, and/or words		

Cursive: *Help peple to do thing.*

Manuscript: *Where are goin*

Figure 24. Types of handwriting errors.

The handwriting problems described above may be characteristic of many low vision print users who do or do not show other learning problems. In identifying remediation techniques, the teacher should keep in mind that writing, spelling, and grammar are each interrelated with the student's articulation and dialect. The essential tool in remediation is to identify each student's most prevalent and unique types of errors and to teach the student to anticipate those errors and avoid them.

A low vision student may have difficulty with the left margin concept in handwriting. The left margin indicates to the beginning reader that a new sentence or thought is to begin. The beginning writer is conditioned to think of sentences beginning on a new line because familiar preprimer books have started each sentence on a new line. Once the string of words that form a sentence is broken by coming back to a new line, the student expects the beginning of a new sentence. The student with learning problems has difficulty expanding the concept that a new line may indicate a beginning of a new sentence or the continuation of a sentence. This means unlearning an earlier learned concept, namely, that each new sentence begins at the left margin. Even when the student has grasped the concept that a new line may begin or continue a sentence in reading, the same student still comes back to the left-hand margin to begin each new handwritten sentence himself. Such problems with margin control are not normal beyond third grade (Mercer & Mercer, 1985).

Students may tend to begin writing in the middle or on the right half of the page rather than starting on the left margin. Their writing may trail down the page toward the right corner. This focusing on the right half of the page may be related to problems involving other tasks which requires the children to attend to objects that cross the midline of the body plane.

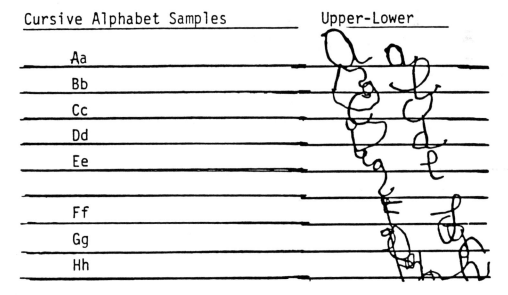

Figure 25. Margin that trails from left to right.

The right margin may be almost totally ignored by a visually impaired student. It is as if the student is attempting to compress each sentence or thought into one writing line. This attempt to fit each sentence on a single line explains why the student will try to compress two or three words into a fraction of an inch at the end of a line, ignoring repeated reminders by the teacher that there is ample space in which to write on the next line. There is such a compulsion to finish a thought on one line that the student may even write on top of words rather than reverting to the left-hand side of the page.

A student with any of the previously described writing habits may retain such writing problems despite repeated teacher interventions which employ techniques and materials available to teach proper letter formation or penmanship. Problems with manuscript writing will probably carry over to cursive writing. The spacing between letters and words, however, may be considerably improved when letters are connected in cursive writing. The teacher may capitalize on the student's new interest and attention in the introduction of cursive writing to make a new start at writing.

Low Vision Teaching Techniques

A structured teaching procedure can be used to develop legible handwriting with students who have problems. A crucial element in this teaching procedure is that the children learn letter formation in three spatial groups: half-line letters, top-line letters, and below-the-line letters. Paper is required with a dotted half-line between the writing line on which the letters rest and the boundary line. The half-line is essential for students to see the three spatially distinct letter groupings, whether they are learning cursive or manuscript.

The pupil should learn the letters by following a written model and the teacher's demonstration. The model can be traced until the correct motor movement is obtained. After much repetition of reproducing or tracing the letters, the pupil should develop a visual and motor model of how the letter is formed. The pupil can then reproduce the letter from looking at the model and by comparing the copy with the model for accuracy as the letter is developed. After some practice, the pupil should be able to reproduce the entire letter from memory and to compare it with the model for accuracy.

Cursive writing has certain unique advantages over manuscript writing for students with either spatial or motor problems. First, since all letters within a word are joined in cursive writing, it is easier for these readers to determine where one word stops and another begins. Second, with the exception for capitals, all cursive letters may begin at the writing baseline. Starting all letters and ending all but four letters (b, w, o,

v) on the line gives students a spatial anchor for the beginning and end of each letter. Third, since cursive handwriting is more adult-like, it is more motivating to students. The following suggestions may be useful for some students with significant problems in cursive handwriting. They may be used collectively with the teaching techniques suggested above or integrated into another handwriting program:

1. Encourage the student to pick up the pencil only at the end of a word or after a capital letter.
2. Check to see that letters fit in the right space: half-line, top-line, or below-the-line.
3. Form letters with as few curves and loops as possible. Teachers can help the pupil with motor problems in handwriting by streamlining letters. The objective is not attractive penmanship but readable handwriting.
4. Allow the student to form "o" and "a" by making a complete circle in only one direction rather than the traditional half-circle and retracing.
5. Discourage multiple attempts to form a letter. The student needs to learn the letter as a kinesthetic whole. Discourage erasing portions of letters or words and rewriting them. When erasing is necessary, encourage erasing the whole word and rewriting it intact.
6. Avoid holding or guiding the student's hand. Guiding the student's hand may be necessary in the beginning instruction stages for every problem writer, but physical help in writing should be faded out as soon as possible.
7. Help the student learn to proof written work by checking with the model. By identifying verbally and in detail their specific problems in forming words, students can be helped to identify and describe differences between the letters they have written and the spatial model. This activity may help to prevent future errors.

Writing rows of a single letter is a beginning technique to practice letter formation. The next step of writing words that include a particular letter may be begun as soon as the student can form several letters. After writing a word several times, the teacher may introduce another word that employs the same letter. If the student repeatedly writes one word or letter, time is insufficient to think about changing from one motor pattern to another. Changing quickly and accurately from one motor pattern to another for each letter is a major component in good handwriting skills. See Figure 26 for a suggested order to cursive letter introduction. The recommended first letters, the half-line letters, the top-line letters, and the below-the-line letters, are introduced after several words have been mastered.

Half-Line Letters	Top-Line Letters	Below-the-Line Letters	Suggested Words With Letter at the		
			Beginning	Middle	End
c					
a	t		at	cat	at
i			it		
	l		lit	ill	tail
e			eat	tell	ice
m			male	came	him
n			name	lane	men
	d		dance	made	and
u			uncle	tune	gnu
r			run	cart	tar
	h		him	the	math
o			out	home	to
s			sit	rash	yes
		g	gone	tagged	drug
w			won	yawn	flew
		y	you	toys	my
	b		but	rubber	cab
	k		kite	bike	kick
		p	pin	tape	stop
		j	jump	major	
		f	fort	sofa	of
x			x-ray	exit	ox
v			vex	lava	
		z	zoo	ozone	whiz
		q	quit	aqua	—

Figure 26. Suggested order of cursive letter introduction.

The most difficult part of cursive writing for many students is not re-membering the motor pattern required to form individual letters but in making a legible transition from one letter to another. Many letter com-binations are quite confusing for visually impaired writers because the joining process is unique. The four letters b, v, w, and o that terminate at the half-line rather than returning to the writing lines pose particular problems. The subsequent letter cannot then be made by starting on the writing line. Students need practice in writing letters after specific words that contain the four problem letters.

Introduce lower-case letters first when teaching either manuscript or cursive writing to visually impaired students. These are the letters that they will be using most for writing and the ones that need the most careful instruction. When upper-case (capital) letters are taught too soon, capital letters may be mixed with lower-case letters within words. Some students may need to continue using capital manuscript letters instead of attempting cursive capitals. This procedure allows the students to practice lower-case cursive without being mentally overloaded by trying to remember the formation of cursive capital letters, too.

The handwriting history of one student who improved his cursive handwriting, using the above described techniques, illustrates the possibilities of special training.

> Matt had completed the first semester in a self-contained fourth grade class of legally blind students at a residential school. Matt's distance visual acuity was measured at 20/200 which is legal blindness. In actual practice he could accurately read sixth grade material printed in 12-point type at 70 words per minute. His main problem in language arts was his poor handwriting skills. When writing in class, Matt always wrote using manuscript unless specifically directed to write cursive. Figure 27 shows samples of Matt's manuscript writing.

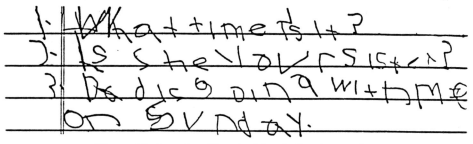

Figure 27. Samples of handwriting before instruction.

The sentences Matt wrote were to read:
1. What time is it?
2. Is she your sister?
3. Dad is going with me on Sunday.

> He received individual help in handwriting for 20 minutes each day. During that time, Matt wrote only in cursive writing. He continued to write with manuscript writing in the classroom for several weeks. Matt was taught each letter as if he were just beginning cursive writing. Matt had been taught most of the upper- and lower-case cursive letters, but he had great trouble remembering the motor patterns. He had spacing inconsistencies within and between words and at times superimposed letters and shifted between letter sizes.

> Matt showed immediate improvement after 3 days in class as he copied from a model with verbal cues from his teacher (see Figure 28). At the end of the school year, Matt was able to compete in an elementary-wide handwriting contest, producing legible cursive writing within the time limit set for his class.

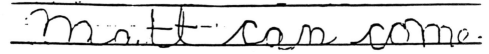

Figure 28. Sample of handwriting after instruction.

To summarize the major guidelines in handwriting instruction for the visually impaired:

1. Introduce the most common and simple letters first.
2. Teach the child letters in groups or pairs that match similar motor movements. Example: (o and a) (i and e).
3. Teach the child how these letters look at the beginning, middle, and end of the word.
4. As early as possible, have the child write actual words.
5. Start with half-line letters and later add top-line letters.
6. Delay letters that hang below the line until last because they are more complex in motor movement.

Signature Writing for Blind Students

Some visually impaired persons may have such limited vision that handwriting is only practical for placing their signatures on legal documents, applications, and checks. These blind persons will find it necessary to learn only the letters required in their names. An example of an informal method that teachers have used successfully is the etching of the signature into a piece of wood and having the blind individual trace the signature until this person learns it well enough to reproduce it using a signature guide over paper. Individual letters can also be traced on wooden blocks (Stocker, 1963). The tracing can also be done over letters which are raised on thermoform sheets. Raised letters can be made on the thermoform machine by using string dipped in Elmer's glue for the impression made on plastic sheets (Freund, 1968).

After demonstrating the shape of a letter on the table from memory, the student should start using a pencil to form the letter on paper. After writing the letter several times, the student should trace the engraved form to check for accuracy. This process should be repeated until the letter can be written in a consistent legible manner (Stark, 1970). After mastering one letter, the student proceeds to the next letter but goes back to review previous letters periodically. After learning all the letters, the student starts putting them together, after first placing the letters in order without connecting them. After learning to connect the letters, an engraved signature is provided for him to trace. Later, after learning to write the signature legibly in large letters, the student learns to gradually reduce the size until the signature can be written within the space on a signature guide (Stark, 1970). The use of raised line paper is helpful in giving the blind person reference points for making the letters.

When writing with either hand, it is recommended that the index finger of the other hand be used to either precede or follow the writing as a place holder (Stark, 1970). For example, in writing with the right hand the left forefinger follows along in the groove between lines as a place holder. When writing with the left hand, the right forefinger precedes the pencil as a place holder.

Several other methods have been introduced to teach letter writing to blind individuals. The "clock" method is one in which the reference points are the positions on a clock face. For example, a "B" is made by starting at 6, going to 3 along the edge of the clock face, then to the center of the clock, back to the 3, then along the edge of the clock face to 12 and then back through the center of the clock to 6. Another method, using the braille cell for orientation of the writer, could be helpful to blind persons who are familiar with braille. The braille cell can be numbered:

    1 . . 4
    2 . . 5
    3 . . 6

A capital "P" would be made by going from dot 3 through dot 2 to dot 1, across to dot 4 and down to dot 5, and back to dot 2 (Weiss & Weiss, 1978). Wheeler (1970) suggested teaching the concept of the diagonal line that is needed in letters such as "K," "M," "V," etc. by using the expanded braille cell on a model or pegboard.

A number of commercial materials are available for use in signature writing instruction. *Longhand Writing for the Blind* (Freund, 1970) consists of a teacher's manual, tracing exercises of letters on plastic thermoform sheets, and a special screen pad and crayon to teach handwriting to blind individuals (See Figure 29). The Marks Writing Guide uses a clipboard with raised metal guidelines to help guide the blind individuals attempting to form letters on a sheet attached to the board (Marks & Marks, 1956). A manual of suggested exercises is included with the board. The Sewell Raised Line Drawing Kit (Weiss & Weiss, 1978) uses a cellophane sheet over a clipboard which has a soft rubber covering. By writing on the cellophane sheet with a ballpoint pen the blind person is enabled to feel the letters which have been cut into the cellophane. Raised line paper, check forms, and signature guides are also commercially available for the blind students.

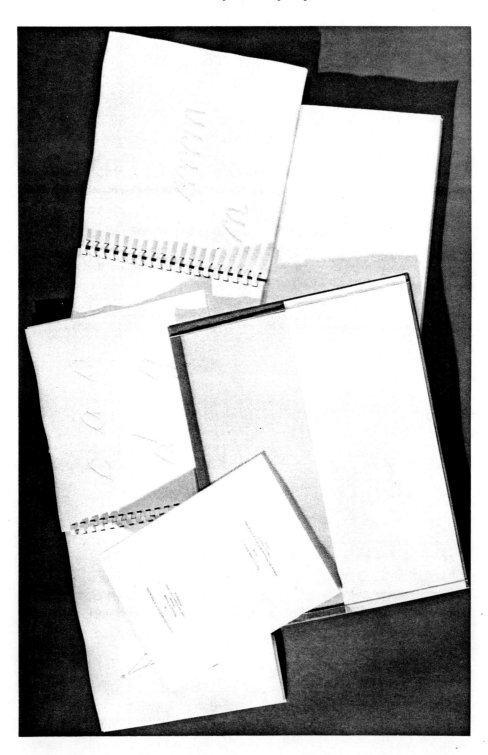

Figure 29. Freund Langland Writing Kit.

Several types of teacher-made materials are sometimes used in signature writing instruction. Tracing this signature with crayon on newsprint paper held over a fine wire screen will help to show the blind person the shapes of the formed letters. Screen pads (Freund, 1968) consist of ordinary window screening stapled to strong paper board. The sides of the pad are bound with masking tape, and a sheet of newsprint paper is fastened to the pad with rubber bands. If an oil crayon is used on the paper the blind student can feel the oily material of the crayon by the many little holes of the underlying mesh. The Arkansas Stringboard is a teacher-made device consisting of a frame with lines of slightly stretched string. Each string has a movable bead which is used as a marker (Weiss & Weiss, 1978).

The blackboard may be a good medium on which to practice early handwriting skills for some children. The blackboard does not move about like paper, and the fine motor movements necessary for handwriting can be practiced (Takemoto, 1964). Tracing and reading letters on monuments in a cemetery is an enrichment exercise that appeals to many blind children. Writing with a stylus into sand or plaster of paris can also show the blind person how he is making the letters.

Raised line paper can also be made by the teacher. Huckins (1965) suggested rolling a sheet of paper tightly around a pencil. After the pencil is removed, the roll is flattened and creased sharply giving lines on the unrolled sheet which are discernible by touch. Raised dot lines can also be made with a slate and stylus or braille writer by embossing parallel rows of dots across the paper. A signature guide can be made by cutting a window in a piece of cardboard. If the blind person has some remaining vision, a closed circuit television can be very useful in helping the person to see the shapes of the letters he has formed while making the letters under the camera of the unit.

Many multihandicapped visually impaired individuals, especially ones with motor problems, may find it extremely difficult to write even under the best circumstances. For these individuals, it may be necessary to use typewriters or microcomputers in order that legible writing can be developed. Special keyboards have been designed that enable motorically handicapped individuals to type even when they have severe motor problems.

BRAILLE WRITING

Writing instruction for low vision students is usually initiated at the preprimer level of reading. As is true of any developmental braille writing process, readiness is an individual matter. Many fine muscle activities are needed to develop the finger strength, coordination, and dexterity necessary for the operation of the braille keys. The child should have sufficient skill to establish correct hand and finger position from the beginning. Bad habits are much more difficult to break than good habits are to form. Ease and fluency in correct fingering are prerequisites to the development of speed and accuracy in writing.

The automatic association of braille dot numbers with the corresponding configuration is useful. If each key on the brailler is identified by a number according to the dot which it forms and each finger is identified by number according to the key it should press, the beginning writer is encouraged to maintain accurate finger position on the keys. The Swing Cell from the American Printing House for the Blind illustrates to the braille student the correspondence between the braille dot number of the vertically aligned dots in the braille cell and the horizontal alignment of the keys of the braille writer (See Figure 30). The dot numbers also provide the best description of any configuration. This description is applicable when referring to the embossed character, to the position of fingers upon the writer keys, or to the formation of symbols with the slate and stylus. The knowledge of dot numbers is a deterrent to the common problem of reversals. Tactual drills in rapid identification of dot numbers determined by their relative positions have been effective in remediation of such problems (Henderson, 1973).

From the first, writing should be a meaningful language process. Alphabet word signs and short-form words offer meaningful configurations for beginners. For example, such forms as "like," "go," "can," and "little," are meaningful, yet they are simple to write. Children are interested in writing their own names. Braille students may start by learning to form their initials, subsequently adding the letters for their entire names.

As the child progresses to writing sentences and short stories, the first focus should be on the expression of ideas rather than on the use of correct contracted forms or fingering of the braille writer keys. As progress in writing continues the teacher may suggest a new way of writing a word; for example, the child may have written "not" in full spelling, and the teacher might suggest a shorter way of writing "not." An examination of the reading book will show the shortened form of "not." An outline of the braille writing skills that may be objectives for instruction at each grade level are in Appendix B: Behavioral Objectives of the Braille Code.

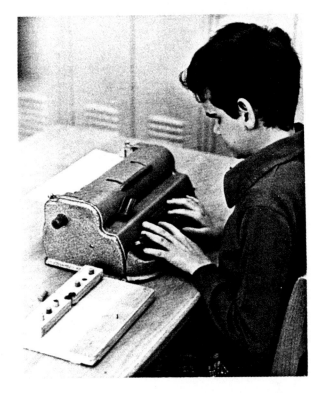

Figure 30. A Perkins Brailler is a good writing machine for children to use. A wooden swing braille cell can be helpful in associating finger position with dot positions.

The Perkins Brailler is useful for most braille students. It can be obtained from Howe Press or by school systems on their quota accounts from the American Printing House for the Blind. The uni-manual brailler is designed for individuals who have use of only one hand. Elongated extension keys are available for individuals with a condition or disability which reduces the amount of pressure that can be exerted on the keys.

The slate and stylus is the most appropriate portable braille writing equipment since it is small, lightweight, and inexpensive. The slate is a hinged metal frame that is closed over the left margin of the paper. Openings in the top section of the frame correspond to the outline of a full, 6-dot braille cell. The bottom section of the frame is a set of depressions for each of the six dots in the cell. The stylus is a slender pointed steel shaft with a rounded point to fit the curvature and elevation of one braille dot (See Figure 31).

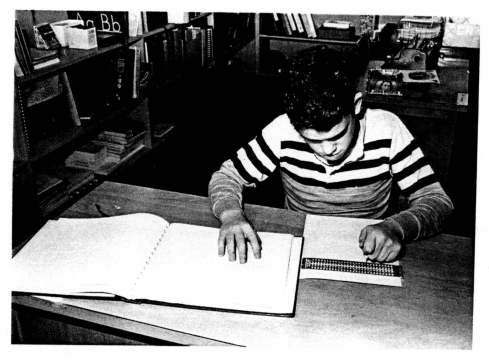

Figure 31. The slate and stylus is small, lightweight, and inexpensive.

Rapid association of dot numbers with braille configurations are beneficial when learning to use the slate and stylus. When writing using a slate and stylus the braille dots are pressed into the paper from the back, thus reversing the material for reading. For this reason, writing begins at the right hand side of the slate and progresses toward the left. When the fingers are moving from left to right reading braille, the first dots encountered are 1, 2, 3, and the next are 4, 5, and 6. The student does not have to form any mental image of the reversed patterns when reading.

The slate should be positioned approximately parallel to the body of the student and on a desk at a height so the arms are parallel to the floor. A slate board to position the paper on the slate is very helpful for beginners and is helpful in the more difficult task of moving the slate down the paper without allowing it to become crooked or writing over previous writing.

Manipulation of the slate and stylus requires much greater hand and finger control than does the operation of the braille. The introduction of the slate and stylus is recommended for the late primary grades when the students have developed a certain level of proficiency in writing with the braille writer. Introduction of the slate and stylus is generally recommended for the third grade level students where students have the prerequisite fine motor skills to emboss the dots. The teacher needs to be careful not to start this fine motor activity before the children are ready. By the sixth grade, students may be expected to take short dictation and complete simple English assignments. A suggested sequence for introducing the slate and stylus is in Appendix B. The time at which the individual will need portable or quiet equipment is also a determining factor. Speed and accuracy in the use of the slate and stylus develop slowly, so this task should be introduced early enough to build efficiency before its use is mandatory. Teachers can encourage the use of the slate and stylus by allowing students to use the lightest weight of paper that will still retain braille of a readable quality.

TYPING SKILLS

The teaching of typing to visually impaired children is very similar to teaching typing to sighted children. Knowledge of the typewriter or computer keyboard is essential to enable visually impaired students to communicate in a written form with sighted teachers and peers. The mechanics of typing should be differentiated from a formal typing curriculum which goes beyond knowledge of the keyboard for touch typing to areas such as the format for friendly letter, business letter, memorandum, and other topics that overlay with an English or language arts curriculum. Almost identical methods and materials are used in their instruction, except that the instructional materials are on a lower grade level since many visually impaired children start typing in the third or fourth grade. However, some differences, especially in adaptations because of visual impairment, may be found useful if adaptations are necessary. The following suggestions might be helpful:

1. When should the student start?

Third or fourth grade is recommended for most visually impaired children (Cohoe, 1961) who do not have multiple handicaps. Some children can start much earlier, but if the child starts too early the necessary finger dexterity and fine muscular coordination may be lacking. For multiply handicapped children who can sit in a chair for 10 minutes, follow a sequence of directions, and have self-help skills such as toilet training established, basic typing skills can be learned in from 2 to 5 years (Dibble, 1984).

2. What are the needed prerequisite skills?

Finger dexterity and muscular control are needed to strike the keys of the keyboard. Dibble (1984) suggested early assessment of hand and finger strengths and appropriate training exercises as needed.

3. What special precautions are recommended?

Good posture is important, especially for visually impaired children. Appropriate reinforcement of good posture and equipment such as special reading stands and easels for holding copy materials are needed. More definite and gradual instruction should be used with visually impaired children (Cohoe, 1961).

4. What special equipment is needed?

Electric pica or bulletin type typewriters are recommended. Cassette recorders with foot pedals to start and stop tapes are helpful for listening to lessons. The Optacon and CCTV can be used to proofread and correct errors.

5. What books and instructional materials are needed?

Most children should be able to use materials for normally seeing children if enlarged, embossed, or recorded on cassette tapes. Most of the typing materials for normally seeing children are on a junior high or high school level. Instructional books on typing for elementary grade children can be purchased in braille, large print, and cassette tapes from the American Printing House for the Blind.

6. What special adaptations are needed?

Special adaptations for visually impaired children include such items as setting margins (Shaw, 1974). The center of the paper can be located by lightly creasing the paper at the center. A tab stop can be set at the center of the paper by locating the crease of the paper after placing the paper in the typewriter. The pupil can backspace from the center point to set margins. Using a backing sheet with a pipestem cleaner attached to the bottom can help to tell the blind typist that the bottom of the paper had been attained. Using a carbon copy can help save material in case "stencil" setting is accidentally set. Using a white wax pencil to mark a place near the bottom of the page can remind the typist to leave space for footnotes (Stark, 1970).

7. Can the new technology in microcomputers be used in teaching typing?

A number of microcomputer programs have been written to teach typing skills to beginning typists. Many visually impaired children will be able to read the regular print from these programs on their monitors. Large print and audio adaptations can be arranged for the low vision and blind students who cannot read the regular print. The advantages of using such programs are motivation and independence for the student.

SUMMARY

Visually impaired children may experience written expression as a natural outgrowth of oral expressions like their normally sighted peers. The major avenues of written expression for visually impaired students are handwriting, braille writing, and typing. Adaptations for teaching handwriting and typing to blind and low vision students are suggested. Suggestions are also made for teaching braille writing through use of the braille writer and the slate and stylus. Although this book focuses largely upon reading instruction, the teacher must remember that reading is only one facet of language and that the development of good writing skills will support and strengthen the reading program. Children, like adults, enjoy reading and having others read materials which they have written themselves. Even though some visually impaired students may not be able to directly read their handwriting and typing, these skills help them communicate with others and may help to build self-esteem as they write like their peers and family members. Developing written expression skills through the medium of writing is a natural part of the language arts curriculum for all students.

CHAPTER 9

THE TEACHING OF LISTENING SKILLS

THE NEED FOR LISTENING SKILLS

AN IMPORTANT trend in special educational programs for visually impaired children is the increasing stress placed on listening as a means of providing information. In 1986, the American Printing House for the Blind listed 23% of its registrants as using listening rather than reading print (36%) or braille materials (15%) (American Printing House, 1986).

The need for listening skills starts in infancy when sound localization enables children to explore their environment, and when sound interpretation helps them to understand object-sound relationships. This development continues into school-age and adulthood when listening provides a means of increasing learning efficiency through substitution for or supplementation of braille and large-type reading materials. Listening activities include listening to recorded books and magazines, listening to teachers, speakers, and friends, and listening to television, radio, microcomputers (with speech output), telephone, calculators, measurement instruments, and electronic devices with speech output.

READINESS FOR LISTENING

Readiness for listening consists of many of the same components as readiness for reading. The following listening skills are among the skills recommended as a foundation to reading (Spache & Spache, 1973):

1. Ability to attend to and recall events in a story
2. Ability to answer simple comprehension questions
3. Ability to follow a sequence in a story

4. Ability to follow simple directions
5. Ability to discriminate sounds
6. Ability to use a listening vocabulary sufficient for concepts in stories
7. Ability to detect similarities and differences in words

Other factors such as intellectual, emotional, social, and physical development are important in the readiness program. Auditory acuity must be considered in listening just as visual acuity is considered in reading print. Auditory acuity is "the ability to detect the presence of sounds at various levels of intensity and frequency and transmit them to the brain" (Oakland & Williams, 1971). Especially important for visually impaired children is concept development. Visually impaired children cannot understand words for which they can attach little meaning because of a lack of experience with the objects represented by the words (Harley, 1963). The chapter on reading readiness refers to some of the problems concerning concept development of visually impaired children.

"Readiness" for listening skills include the components of auditory training. Sequencing the components of auditory perception can be very helpful to the teacher of visually impaired children. Langley (1986) has developed a very useful table of developmental tasks for screening auditory function from birth to school-age, showing test items, procedure, developmental level response, and nonverbal sound. A hierarchy of these components is suggested by Heasley (1974):

1. Awareness of sound
2. Auditory attending
3. Auditory attention span
4. Sound localization
5. Auditory discrimination
6. Auditory memory
7. Auditory memory span
8. Auditory sequencing ability
9. Auditory projection ability
10. Auditory figure-ground discrimination
11. Auditory blending
12. Auditory clozure
13. Re-auditorization

Awareness of Sound

Auditory awareness is noted by the ability of the child to change behavior by the presence or absence of sound (Heasley, 1974). Does the child startle, stop or start crying, or react in any other way in response to sound? Voices or environmental sounds are sounds that even infants will react to almost from birth. In the classroom, the teacher might use a tape of environmental sounds or informal observations to see if the child reacts to any of these sounds. If the child has a hearing problem, sound may need to be amplified in order that the child can hear the sound. Even a child cognitively unable to interpret sounds can show a startle reaction to sounds if the hearing mechanism is intact and able to send signals to the brain.

Auditory Attenting

Auditory attenting is the intention to listen or accept responsibility for processing language or non-language sound stimuli (Heasley, 1974). The child who is attending auditorily not only is aware of the sound but also tunes in to the sound. An auditory selection test to measure attention to environmental noises is a part of the Goldman-Fristoe-Woodcock Test Battery.

Auditory Attention Span

Auditory attending is the child's ability to attend selectively to language or non-language sounds for increased periods of time. If the child is motivated, the teacher should be able to increase the child's attention span over a period of time with auditory perceptual exercises. Maintenance of records with the use of good auditory materials on the child's level should help to increase auditory attention span.

Sound Localizaton

Localizaton of sound requires the location of the direction from which a language or non-language sound originated. Visually impaired infants will have considerable difficulty in moving about within their environments without learning sound localization. Warren (1984) found no evidence to indicate that visual impairment creates a handicap in any of the basic auditory discriminative abilities of loudness, sound quality, or pitch. However, reaching to an object by sound alone was found to occur much later than reaching for objects by sight (Fraiberg, Siegel, & Gibson, 1966). Sound is extremely important to blind infants in developing sound-object relationship. If blind infants don't associate sound with an object they may not have any reason to move out into the environment toward these sound-making objects. This means that sighted infants have visual stimuli to prompt them to reach out and explore objects in their environment as much as several months before visually impaired children are prompted by sound stimuli to explore.

The Peabody Mobility Kit for Infants and Toddlers is designed with a section on sound localization (Harley & Long, 1986). The training activities are step-by-step guides to helping young, multihandicapped blind children acquire fundamental skills which provide a base for independent movement. A very fine-grained sequence of activities moves from an awareness of sounds level to a final level in which the child can locate a sound-making object several feet away from the child.

Auditory Discrimination

Auditory discrimination is the ability to recognize and respond appropriately to similarities and differences in language or non-language sounds. Auditory discrimination can usually be tested by simple adaptations of tests which are used with normally seeing children. The Auditory Discrimination Test (Wepman, 1973) is one of the most commonly used tests of auditory discrimination with young blind children. This test, which has norms ranging from ages 5-8, does not require visual ability. The test measures the ability to hear accurately the differences which exist between the phonemes used in English speech. The child is asked to listen to pairs of words that are the same word or differ by only one phoneme and to indicate similarity or difference. Administration of the test to older 5-year-old children and younger 6-year-olds permits the selection of those who are likely to have difficulty learning to use the phonics necessary for reading. For older children, it has been found to be helpful in diagnosis of reading difficulties.

Auditory Memory

Auditory memory is the ability to store and recall auditory material (Northern & Downs, 1974) such as a sound or series of language or non-language sounds. If the learner cannot remember certain sounds, it would be difficult to associate an object with the sound or to interpret the meaning of the sound. Then, the child should be able to remember the object-sound relationship and be able to understand and make discoveries by locating sounds and moving toward them. A sequence of three commands is given to remember in the Detroit Tests of Learning Aptitude-Oral Directions and Oral Commissions (Northern & Downs, 1974).

Auditory Memory Span

Auditory memory span refers to an individual's ability to remember over increasing lengths of time the nature or characteristics of a sound (Heasley, 1974). For example, the child is told about the sound of running water in a water faucet when it is turned on. After learning the meaning of the sound, the child recalls what the water faucet sound means when the child hears it again. Environmental sound tapes can be made by the teacher or purchased commercially to increase auditory memory span. Auditory memory span could also apply to the remembering over time of verbal commands.

Auditory Sequencing Ability

The ability to remember the order of items in a sequence of language or non-language sounds may be called auditory sequencing ability (Northern & Downs, 1974). An example of such sequencing occurs when the child recalls "Mamma goes" after "Mamma goes to the store" is spoken. The Goldman-Fristoe-Woodcock Auditory Skills Test Battery consists of three memory tests: recognition memory, memory for content, and memory for sequence. This test relies heavily on pictures and may need to be adapted with blind and some low vision children. Some studies have shown that blind children tend to score higher on auditory sequential memory subtests, such as digit span, than normally seeing children (Smits & Mommers, 1976). In this test, children are asked to repeat numbers like "1-4" and increasing to "2-8-9," etc. An example of this procedure is the digit span test on the Wechsler Intelligence Scale for Children (Bortner, 1985) or sentence memory on the Brigance Diagnostic Inventory of Basic Skills (Witt, 1985).

Auditory Projection

Auditory projection may be defined as the ability of the visually impaired child to attend to and interpret language or non-language sounds which come from a distance (Heasley, 1974). Some children are only able to attend to and to process sounds which are in the immediate vicinity. The teacher can help the child to listen at increasingly greater distances. A related skill of voice projection has been identified as a problem for visually impaired persons. Cutsforth (1951) describes the "broadcasting voice" as a problem with some blind individuals.

Auditory Figure-Ground Discrimination

Auditory separation is comparable to the visual skill of figure-ground discrimination. It is the child's ability to attend to a particular sound or series of sounds when other competing sounds are also present (Heasley, 1974). It is like listening to mother's instructions while the radio or TV set is playing in the same room. The child may be unable to attend to mother in the presence of the competing TV distraction. The Goldman-Fristoe-Woodcock Auditory Skills Test has a subtest on auditory selective attention in which the listener must ignore distracting background noises which become increasingly intense.

Auditory Blending

Auditory blending is the child's ability to blend speech sounds. It is sometimes described as the ability to synthesize isolated phonemic sounds into a whole word (Northern & Downs, 1974). Goldman, Fristoe, & Woodcock (1974) have developed a test which includes a subtest for auditory blending ability. The Diagnostic Reading Scales (Spache 1972) also includes a phoneme blending subtest as do various other diagnostic reading tests. This subtest would be particularly useful in determining problems that children might have in phonics instruction.

Auditory Clozure

Auditory clozure is the ability to identify the true or accurate pronunciation of a word. It is sometimes defined as the ability to synthesize some of the separate sounds of a word into a whole word (sometimes called auditory interaction) (Heasley, 1974). In the Illinois Test of Psycholinguistic Abilities, auditory clozure consists of having the child supply a completed word from an incomplete stimulus word (e.g., "Daddy" from "Day").

Re-Auditorization

Re-auditorization is the unvoiced recollection and holding of a sound production (Heasley, 1974). This recollection is important in speech development. If infants imitate an inflection pattern heard from their mothers, they must remember and hold for reference for future reproduction the sound characteristics of the signal.

Exercises for developing efficiency in the preceding component areas of auditory perception can be found in *Auditory Perception Disrorders and Remediation* by Heasley (1974). Assessment instruments which have items for measuring auditory skills include the Bayley Scales of Infant Development, the Brigance Diagnostic Inventory of Early Development, the Hauserman Scale of Developmental Potential of Preschool Children, the Koontz Child Development Program, and the Learning Accomplishment Profile.

THE TEACHING OF LISTENING SKILLS

Lundstein (1979, p. 1) defines listening as "The process by which spoken language is converted to meaning in the mind." Listening is often compared to reading. In both processes, symbols are converted to meaning. In both processes, the concepts representing words must be understood in order to convey meaning. Listening vocabulary for children is usually more expansive than speaking vocabulary, and the speaking vocabulary is more comprehensive than the reading vocabulary. The listening comprehension skills such as selecting facts and details, sequential ordering, selecting main idea, summarizing, making inferences, etc. are the same skills that are needed in reading comprehension.

There are many kinds of listening activities. Smith (1972) groups these various kinds of listening activities into four categories: attentive, analytical, appreciative, and marginal. *Attentive listening* is defined as listening in which attention is focused on one person or one form of communication, such as a telephone conversation or a radio broadcast. *Analytical listening* is attentive listening plus giving a response requiring analysis or thinking carefully about what the speaker is saying, such as drawing inferences or identifying a sequence of events. *Appreciative listening* is the type of listening in which one listens to music, poetry, or stories being read. *Marginal listening* is the kind of listening in which there are two or more distractions present, such as listening to music while painting or writing creatively. Another type of listening is *selective listening* or listening to certain sounds while screening out other distractions.

Most of the literature on listening for the visually impaired deals with analytical listening. In order to understand analytical listening, Lundstein (1979) devised a listening taxonomy which starts with prerequisite sound identification skills and proceeds to one of the most difficult of the analytical skills, inference making. The following hierarchical objectives would be appropriate for teaching listening skills to children up to the middle grades of school:

1. Discriminates and identifies verbal and nonverbal sounds
2. Demonstrates listener-speaker responsibility
3. Recalls facts and details
4. Identifies sequential order
5. Selects main idea
6. Summarizes
7. Relates one idea to another
8. Makes inferences

Other kinds of analytical listening skills that may be included are: finds emotional persuasion, draws comparisons, makes judgments, recognizes stated cause and effect relationships, draws conclusions, makes generalizations, recognizes purpose, determines accuracy of information, differentiates fact from opinion, discounts bias of speaker, recognizes propaganda techniques, finds hidden purpose, solves problems, and predicts outcomes (Burns, 1980). The teacher of visually impaired children should consult a book on listening or communication skills to learn more about the teaching of listening skills, such as Adventures in Communication by James A. Smith (1972) or Assessment and Correction of Language Arts Difficulties by Paul C. Burns (1980).

Measurement of Analytical Listening Ability

The measurement of analytical listening skills may be obtained informally, using teacher-made criterion-referenced tests in which the teacher makes up her own comprehension questions. For example, the teacher reads to the child a selection from a reading book and then asks the child to recall facts and details, to choose the main idea, or to put events in sequential order. Criterion-referenced tests will help the teacher to make short-range instructional decisions and to see how well the child's instructional objectives are being achieved. Measurement of listening skills can also be obtained through the use of standardized tests (see Figure 32).

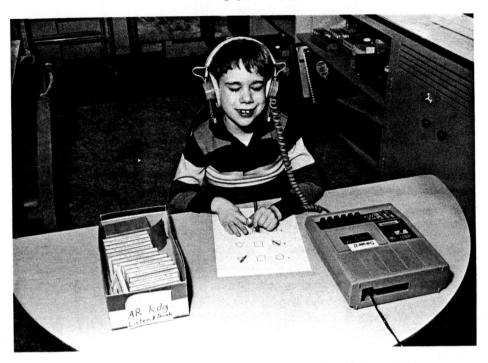

Figure 32. Listening may be evaluated, using formal and informal measures.

The Stanford Achievement Test: Listening Comprehension Tests (Levels Primary 2 through Advanced) are designed for grades 1.5 to 9.9. After each passage, the examiner reads from one to four comprehension questions presented in multiple choice format. The answer booklets which use pictured options up through the first part of Primary 2 (Schutz, 1985) may need to be adapted for visually impaired learners. Beyond the Primary 2 or second grade level, the response choices in the booklet are words or phrases. The examiner reads both the passage and the possible choices so that reading skills are not required. This test is available in braille and large print from the American Printing House.

The Sequential Tests of Educational Progress (STEP), designed for grades 4-14, provides a subtest that measures analytical listening abilities, such as comprehending main ideas, remembering significant details, and understanding implication of the ideas and details. Norms for blind children in grades 4, 5, and 6 are available (Pearson, 1963). This test provides grade equivalencies, scaled scores, and percentiles for sighted norms and for the blind is available in braille and large print from the American Printing House. The Durrell Listening-Reading Series (Wood, 1981) also in braille and large print may be used to compare the child's reading ability with his listening ability in grades 1-9. The purposes of these tests are to identify children with reading problems and to measure the degree of retardation in reading to listening ability. The listening comprehension, as measured on the vocabulary and paragraph meaning sections, is designed to show the child's intellectual and perceptual ability to handle words and sentences as a basis for reading instruction.

The SRA Achievement Series has subtests in auditory discrimination and listening comprehension that can be used in grades K-12. Other sections of this test can be read orally to the pupil, and the accompanying comprehension questions can be used to check for listening skills.

The Educational Testing Service provides listening subtests in the Cooperative Primary Tests for grades 1-3. The teacher reads words, sentences, stories, and expositions, and the child demonstrates comprehension by marking appropriate pictures. The assessed skills include identifying illustrative or associated instances, recalling elements, interpreting the presented ideas, and drawing inferences (Lundstein, 1979).

Checklists can be very helpful to the teacher in assessing listening. Furness (1955) devised such a checklist that has been reproduced in a number of books on the teaching of listening skills. The 13 categories include the following:

1. Physiological (faculty auditory discrimination)
2. Speech problems
3. Fatigue
4. Physical discomfort
5. Psychological (lack of listening readiness)
6. Emotional maladjustments
7. Personality traits
8. Retarded mental development
9. Lack of interest in material
10. Lack of purpose
11. Half-listening (poor listening habits)
12. Failure to listen discriminatively
13. Failure to listen critically

Each disability is matched by a list of possible causes and suggested teaching procedures.

An informal reading inventory may be used to measure listening comprehension of prose passages (Hargrove & Poteet, 1984). After passages from readers are read aloud to the student, related comprehension questions are asked. Testing with more difficult passages continues until the student's accuracy falls below 75%. The appropriate listening level is the level at which the student is able to just answer 75% of the questions.

Nolan and Morris (1973) found that intelligence, grade level, and ability to read braille are factors which affect learning through listening. The more intelligent and higher grade level pupils did better in listening than the less intelligent and lower grade level pupils. The braille readers often obtained higher comprehension scores than large type readers. They attributed this difference partially to differences in mental ability of the groups and partially to the greater necessity of braille readers to rely on listening as a source of information.

THE NEED FOR LISTENING SKILLS

The demand for listening materials is indicated by the many books and magazines that are readily available on tape from commercial publishers. In addition, the demand is shown by special agencies serving visually impaired persons to provide listening materials free or at nominal costs. These agencies are:

1. National Library Service (periodicals, books, talking book machine, cassette players)
2. American Printing House for the Blind (textbooks, instructional materials)
3. Recordings for the Blind, Inc. (school and college textbooks)

In addition, local public libraries and radio reading services for the blind are sources of books in recorded form.

Listening has proven to be an effective means of providing information for the following groups of listeners:

1. Visually Impaired Adults. The National Library Service for the Blind and Physically Handicapped (1986) indicated that listening materials are by far the most popular for the adults who lose vision in adulthood and have not acquired effective braille reading skills. The policy of this federal agency is to produce as much materials as possible in recorded format so that all of their constituents can use it. Mack (1984) found that the majority of 30 blind adults in California who had learned

and used braille as their primary reading mode in public schools reported using braille only for personal notes and memoranda. However, they relied on readers and recordings for most of their reading. The blind adults reported disadvantages of braille as (a) slowness in reading (50%), (b) takes up too much space (27%), and (c) unavailability of materials in braille (27%).

2. Visually Impaired College Students. Readers, talking books, and tape recorders are needed by college students. Braille and large-print copies of college texts are almost nonexistent, and information processing is much faster with listening.

3. Visually Impaired Multihandicapped Children. Nolan and Kederis (1969) recommended listening over braille reading for pupils below an Intelligent Quotient of 85. Steele (1969) found that blind children with IQs below 85 learned more from listening when their reading comprehension in braille was low.

4. Visually Impaired Preschool Children. Visually impaired preschool children, including infants and toddlers, need to develop listening skills for better communication with their environments. Instructional programs in sound localization for visually impaired infants and toddlers have been developed and validated. (Harley & Long, 1986).

5. Visually Impaired School-Age Pupils. Listening for some children may be more efficient than either braille or large print reading. The teacher of visually impaired children will soon find that the reading rates of her children are quite slow. An exception would be mathematical and scientific materials employing formulas and tables; they may be easier to comprehend in braille or large print.

Listening has gained more interest by teachers of school-age visually impaired children and youth, not only because of increased availability of recorded materials, but because of the increased learning efficiency of listening over large type and braille reading materials for many students. The popularity of listening is easy to understand when children read braille and print materials at very slow rates of speed. The average blind high school senior reads braille at about 86 words per minute (Ethington, 1956), and legally blind large type secondary school students read print at about 90 words per minute (Nolan, 1959). Talking books and other recorded materials provide speeds of about 175 words per minute (Nolan & Morris, 1973). Nolan (1963), using braille reading subjects from grades 6-10, found that information could be obtained through listening in one third of the braille reading time without loss of comprehension. Morris (1966) found that learning through listening appeared to be 155-360% more efficient than learning through reading in braille or large type with legally blind subjects from grades 4-6 and high school.

An analysis of the reading-listening efficiency studies show that the relative superiority of listening over braille or large print is contingent upon reading rate. For example, a study by Nolan (1963) showed that comprehension of the listening subjects did not differ from that of the braille reading subjects. However, the listening group expended less time in listening than in reading, making listening more efficient. Wood (1981), using the Durrell Listening-Reading series with 71 visually impaired children from the grades 4-6, found that listening comprehension was superior to braille and print reading comprehension at each grade level even when reading times were longer than the listening times of the subjects. However, a limit was placed on the reading time, and poorer readers did not have sufficient time to finish the selected exercises.

Listening materials may be specifically prepared for visually impaired persons or used from regular publishers. The American Printing House for the Blind has adapted a series of tapes to train listening skills called Listen and Think (see Figure 32). The sets of tapes are in levels starting with auditory readiness. Each level contains approximately 15 tapes. Each tape focuses on a different purpose of listening such as recognizing cause and effect, main idea, classifying, and inferring.

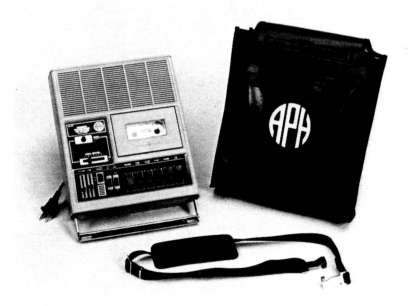

Figure 33. This cassette tape recorder and player is especially designed for visually impaired persons. Courtesy of the American Printing House for the Blind.

Other materials from the American Printing House that are accessable through listening include a dictionary and tutorials in a variety of subjects including cell division, map reading, typing, and microbiology.

The increased use of the microcomputer with a speech synthesizer has added new dimensions to the purposes of listening. The importance of listening in using word processing programs as writing tools is an emerging area of listening.

THE IMPROVEMENT OF LISTENING COMPREHENSION

How does one improve the listening comprehension of visually impaired persons? Two general methods have been reported in the research literature. One method of improving analytical listening skills is to train the listener through special instruction. Active listening helps to improve listening (Nolan & Morris, 1969). The listener who takes notes, asks questions of a speaker, and controls the speed of the taped materials, tends to do much better in listening than the passive listener. Pupils who use well-organized listening techniques score highest academically (Carter, 1962). Bischoff (1967) found that listening skills can be improved by special instruction, using sequential listening comprehension lessons graduated in length and complexity. He divided 63 low vision pupils from grades 4-9 into two experimental groups and one control group. Each experimental group received two 15-minute listening lessons per week for 10 weeks, one from My Weekly Reader listening comprehension paragraphs and the other from SRA listening lessons. The experimental group which received listening comprehension lessons increased in listening efficiency, but the control group actually showed a decrease. Bischoff (1979) suggested an upright posture and elimination of outside distractions to improve listening comprehension. Teachers should become aware that listening efficiency could be improved by instruction and that with increased listening efficiency recorded materials could better supplement reading materials in the classroom.

An extensive programmatic research study of aural systems for the visually handicapped has been undertaken at the American Printing House for the Blind to study the process of learning through listening and to develop system-playback equipment, textbook formats, and study techniques designed for this purpose (Nolan & Morris, 1973). Among the general findings have been that intelligence and grade level correlate positively with listening comprehension. High school children profit more from repeated listening presentations than elementary level children. High school students profit more from mass exposure to listening presentations than elementary students, who do better under distributed presentations over time. Length of attention span was postulated as the cause of differences between the two groups.

Nolan & Morris (1969) found that segmenting of a message does not enhance listening comprehension if total time on task is held constant, and giving a prior summary of the message before the presentation does not aid comprehension for legally blind students in grades 4-12. Comprehension was best with notetaking, and lowest with continuous listening. Active participation led to greater learning for literature, science and social studies at the high school level. Active participation consisted of mental review, notetaking, and discussion of tape materials.

A second method which has received increased attention is one of improving the instructional package. Methods with sighted subjects have included the use of telegraphic prose, humorous stories, visual image, and listening patterns with active involvement of the listener. Morris (1976a), in a series of studies for facilitating listening as a medium for education of the visually impaired, compared the use of indexing systems to determine if use of recorded reference materials is feasible and desirable for persons who are visually handicapped. The disc indexing system consisted of written material, a unique record format with separation bands, page numbers and word cues, and a special record player with variable speed capability. This system was tested with 36 braille and large print subjects in grades 4-12. Later, a cassette system was evaluated with 24 braille and large type subjects from grades 7-12 to test their skill at locating entries in a recorded form from an encyclopedia. The indexed cassette player was designed with tone index points which could be found quickly with a high speed pulse counting network. The results indicated that blind students could use the cassette reference system with an acceptable degree of accuracy and within appropriate time constraints. In a consumer survey teachers, librarians, and blind students preferred having index information for a dictionary superimposed at a higher speed on the same track with the content or having index information on the track running parallel to the content tack (Morris & Hill, 1976). Cobb (1977) designed a two-track indexed tape with one channel for exposition with questions and a second channel of commentary with review questions. An advantage of learning with such tapes is that students can be more active in responding to the tape recorded material.

THE IMPROVEMENT OF LISTENING SPEED

The speed of information processing attained by listening at approximately 175 words per minute is relatively slow when considering the speed of reading attained by sighted high school and college students. For this reason, much effort has been focused on increasing the speed of aural materials. Accelerated or compressed speech can be used to speed up information processing by listening. Popular methods of accelerating speech include (1) speaking rapidly, (2) increasing the play back speed of tape or record, and (3) sampling segments of the speech signal. Speaking rapidly is limited since only a moderate increase in rate of articulation of speech sound by the speaker is possible. Increasing the speed of a tape or record results in a higher pitch, making intelligibility difficult at high speeds. A pitch restorer that electronically returns the pitch to the original range can be secured from the American Printing House for the Blind.

The research studies have been concerned primarily with intelligibility and comprehension of accelerated speech materials produced by various methods and the characteristics and training of the listeners. For example, compression beyond 275 words per minute has resulted in a sharp decline in retention of information (Foulke, 1966). Nolan & Morris (1969) reported that high school students learned significantly more at 175 words per minute than at 225 words per minute.

Tuttle (1972) compared reading by listening at normally recorded speed and reading by listening to compressed speech with a sample of braille readers from 14-21 years of age. After each subject took three equivalent forms of a prose reading test, he found no difference in comprehension among the three reading media. However, braille reading took almost twice as long as reading by listening to compressed speech and oral speech, using the Durrell Reading-Listening Test with 41 visually impaired subjects.

SUMMARY

Listening is important to visually impaired learners from infancy through adulthood. A major conclusion that could be drawn from the research with visually impaired children is that learning by listening is generally more efficient than learning from braille and large type reading when the important factor of time is considered. The evidence also indicates that listening efficiency can be improved by instruction and by adapting the design of the listening materials and playback equipment to suit the individual abilities of the visually impaired learner.

CHAPTER 10

BRAILLE READING FOR THE LATE BLINDED

LATE BLINDED youths or adults may want to read and write braille for a variety of reasons. They may wish to read books or magazines for entertainment, information, hobbies, education, religion, general instruction, news, or public affairs. They may only desire to learn a simple braille code that would enable them to read labels and phone numbers. They soon learn that information from many books and magazines is also available on talking book records and cassette or open-reel tapes through the United States Library of Congress, the American Printing House for the Blind, Recordings for the Blind, and other volunteer sources such as Radio Reading Services. They also learn that sighted readers are available for many blind persons, and some blind people have access to books and magazines through new electronic devices, such as the cassette or optical reader with a speech synthesizer.

READINESS FOR BRAILLE READING

Certain considerations are unique to the learning situation for the individuals who have previously read print but who find it necessary to learn braille as a new means of communication. These characteristics are discussed and possible materials are suggested in the following section. Suggestions for newly blinded children, as well as youth and adults, are presented. The beginning youth and adult will need a braille readiness program just as the beginning young blind child needs a readiness program before starting to read braille. Important factors to consider in designing a readiness program are the following:

1. Emotional readiness
2. Perceptual readiness
3. Academic readiness

Emotional Readiness

Late blinded youths and adults who must change from print to braille as their medium of reading may be experiencing some emotional adjustment that will affect their ability to learn braille. Very young children who enter school with insufficient vision to read print will more likely approach reading through braille with the natural thrill of learning to read. On the other hand, those print readers who must change from print to braille may have a negative approach to reading. They may have negative attitudes toward their visual impairment because of the attitude of their family and friends. They may have already experienced failure in reading. Some may have been only marginal print readers. The teacher must provide adequate motivation and sufficient positive reinforcement to overcome these negative feelings.

A negative feeling towards blindness may be especially strong for the individuals who have suffered the traumatic experience of sudden blindness resulting in total dependence upon their other senses. The individuals who are in the process of adjusting to blindness may vary from day to day in their readiness for their braille lessons. For example, one high school girl who had suffered loss of vision frequently came to her braille lesson and seemed unable to concentrate on her work. Ordinarily, she was a good student. Investigation revealed that on her *off days* she was angry with herself and upset over her blindness because she had become lost on the school grounds on which she had been totally familiar as a sighted person. If braille had been required on these off days, she could have developed a poor attitude toward this new medium.

Visually impaired youths or adults will have little success in mastering braille if they have not yet made positive adjustments to blindness. Some pupils fail to learn to read braille because they associate braille as a symbol of their blindness that they have not fully accepted. They may fail to accept themselves as blind persons because of negative attitudes toward blindness that they shared as a sighted person. Cholden (1958) suggested that newly blinded individuals must go through shock and depression stages before accepting themselves as handicapped persons. They must realize that they have lost a part of themselves and that they are now new persons with different capacities and potentials. Until they reach this point of adjustment, it is useless to attempt to teach them braille or any other skill associated with blindness. During the shock and depression stages, counseling is needed rather than a teaching program. When the newly blinded individuals finally accept themselves as blind persons, they are ready for learning new communications skills such as braille reading.

Perceptual Readiness

The late blinded need a different kind of readiness program than young blind children. The major kind of readiness needed is tactual-kinesthetic readiness. Most potential readers can start by learning to discriminate geometric dot patterns. Later, they proceed to trace lines of braille cell patterns and to discriminate different symbols within a line. The *Touch and Tell* series (Duncan, 1969) from the American Printing House for the Blind or the *Kansas Braille Reading-Readiness Book of Modern Methods of Teaching Braille* (Stocker, 1970) can be used for this purpose. The Tactual Discrimination Worksheets from the American Printing House were successfully used by the 37-65 year old diabetic adults in a study of tactually impaired blind beginning braille readers (Harley, Pichert, & Morrison, 1985).

A braille readiness program by Billie Elder (Weiss, 1980) was used successfully with blind adults at Arkansas Enterprises for the Blind. The exercises in this program begin with lines of varying braille patterns in order to teach the learner a horizontal reading pattern while using both hands. A second component of this program trains the learner to discriminate between similar and dissimilar tactile patterns on cards. A deck of playing cards may be embossed with the appropriate braille dots and used with beginners to sharpen recognition of braille cell patterns. The advantage of using brailled playing cards is the motivation to play a game. Many adults can move to braille cell discrimination exercises almost immediately since their tactual perceptual skills have already been well-developed.

Associated with the loss of vision may be medical, physiological, or neurological conditions that may also lessen tactual sensitivity. For example, an accident victim who has had a injury to the head may have a mild neurological impairment causing a decrease in tactual sensitivity. For the diabetic, tactual perception varies greatly from day to day. The ability to perceive through the fingertips should be assessed and developed through readiness activities. Some typical activities are found on the initial pages of *ABC's of Braille* (Krebs, 1973). Teacher-prepared materials in which the individual is asked to locate the symbol which is different or to locate two symbols which are the same can be used to assess ability as well as to alert the learner to the differential characteristics

within the braille code. The reader is asked to detect differences in the
following:

1. A line of braille characters in which only one character is different
   where the differentiation depends on the absence of only one dot, for
   example, all "p,s" except for one "s."

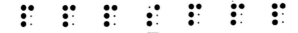

2. A row of characters in which the differentiation depends only on left-
   right alignment. For example, a row of "k's" with only one dot 4-6.

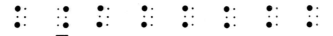

3. A row of characters that requires spatial differentiation in several
   fields. For example, finding the two like symbols existing in a row including "b u," 2-3 "u," and two items of 4-5 "u."

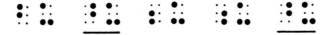

The development of tactual discrimination skills is needed by newly
blinded adults who have relied primarily on visual skills for reading
print. Stocker and Walton (1967) recommended two weeks of readiness
exercise before the introduction of braille. For example, left to right
movement and staying on the line were stressed. In addition, the development of tactual perceptual abilities through following a sequential
step-by-step program which proceeds from gross to fine patterns was
recommended.

The *Kansas Braille Reading Readiness book* (Stocker, 1970) has been
used with blind adults. The following exercises are designed to build
readiness skills:

1. The use of both hands in tactual discrimination of shapes and sizes of
   geometric figures
2. Left to right movement in tracing a line and returning to the next
   line
3. Holding the fingers so that all dots can be read

4. Tactual discrimination of braille cells to refine spatial concepts, kinesthetic memory, and discrimination abilities.

The second volume of this series provides exercises in learning Grade 2 braille. The close spacing between lines without guidelines may be troublesome to some beginning readers.

Academic Readiness

The teacher who is attempting to help late blinded individuals to read braille needs some insight into their academic backgrounds. Frequently, the students' learning problems become more noticeable when they reach junior high or high school levels. Since their visual difficulty is obvious it is assumed to be the cause of any learning problems, and the visually impaired students are referred for instruction in braille. Diagnosis often reveals that visual difficulty is only one aspect of a larger disability. Too frequently, such students have been excused from essential classroom learning activities. They have been passed along with good academic grades under the rationalization that they should not be penalized for poor vision. Finally, the late blind students reach the critical period when they must change to braille, but they have no foundation of word-attack skills or of comprehension skills. The teacher who fails to diagnose this deficiency may spend a great deal of time and effort in teaching the braille words only to discover that the students can recognize and spell words without being able to pronounce them. They may identify all the words in a sentence or paragraph without being able to understand the meaning. Instruction would have been much more effective if the teacher had taught *reading* as the primary goal, developing knowledge of the braille code more gradually as the work progressed.

Several measures can be utilized to assess the academic background of the pupil. An oral spelling test gives a good clue to phonic ability. A list such as the spelling section of the Wide Range Achievement Test is appropriate for testing this ability. However, any graded spelling list is adequate if it includes words at increasing levels of difficulty. The purpose of this measure is not to assign a specific grade level of functioning, or to measure absolute accuracy in spelling, but to determine the phonetical accuracy of the student's spelling. If the spelling words are attacked phonetically, the student will probably be able to do the same in reading.

Comprehension or interpretive skills may be measured by means of a test in listening comprehension, such as the procedure suggested in the Spache Diagnostic Reading Scales. A very informal assessment can be obtained by reading to the student a textbook passage and asking questions requiring interpretation. When the cloze technique is used as a measure of comprehension, the teacher reads a sentence containing a significant missing word, and the student is asked to give the missing word. Any sensible response indicates adequate use of context clues. Good examples of such sentences can be found in "Using the Context" out of the Specific Skill Series. In using these sentences, the teacher allows students to supply their own words without giving the multiple choice examples. A more extensive description of the assessment of academic skill levels may be found in Chapter 5, Assessment of Reading Skills.

Most adventitiously blind adults only need braille reading or another type of embossed system for daily living skills. They can read books and magazines more efficiently through the use of recorded media. The Fishburne alphabet can be used for reading labels on food containers and medicine bottles or for reading telephone numbers (Newman & Hall, 1986).

Many adventitiously blind children and adults will not need to learn braille. Optical aids such as head-born, hand-held, or stand magnifiers, closed circuit television, and telescopes can be used to help them read and travel more easily. Large print books will be helpful to some, and some may want to learn braille. There are several levels of embossed dot and braille reading that could be useful in devising objectives for these adults. These levels begin at the easiest level and proceed to the most difficult levels:

1. Reading dots on watches, thermostats, electrical appliances, measuring devices, etc. (See Figure 34)
2. Reading numbers on elevators, bingo and playing cards, and other games
3. Reading labels on medicine, food, and clothing items
4. Reading telephone numbers and addresses
5. Reading menus, recipes, and instructions on equipment
6. Writing letters, keeping a diary, record of personal expenses
7. Reading short stories and words to music in Grade 1
8. Reading books in Grade 2 braille, taking notes in class
9. Using computers and paperless braille recorders (Grade 1 and Grade 2 braille)

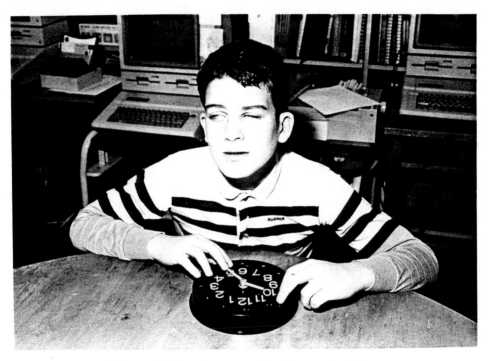

Figure 34. Learning to read braille on a clock face.

METHODS AND MATERIALS

For children who must change from print to braille during the primary grades, the best approach is probably the braille modification of the instructional method used with them in print reading. If the children enjoyed the stories in print, they would probably enjoy similar stories or the same stories in braille. Previous acquaintance with stories should help students read quickly.

Stories in rhyme which can be found on the early level of many library books or braille editions of juvenile periodicals encourage fluent reading because the child begins to grasp the rhyming stories by memory and the fingers move quickly. Stories composed by the child or about the child's experiences also provide good reading material. Familiarity with the content helps the fingers to move quickly, and the student has an important feeling of success. Reader's Digest Reading Skill Builders contain stories with mature content on beginning reading levels and are available in braille from the American Printing House for the Blind.

For students changing to braille during the upper elementary or secondary levels, a manual may serve as the core for instruction. A popular manual, *ABC's of Braille* by Bernard Krebs (1973), introduces the braille code. Once students have a good start, they can use this manual to work at their own speed. However, adjustments must be made to meet individual needs. There are sections in this manual in which the student will probably need additional learning time and practice materials. *Braille in Brief* by Krebs (1968) presents a very similar program to the *ABC's of Braille.* Another set of materials designed to teach braille to newly blinded persons who have already read print is *Read Again* from the American Printing House for the Blind. The materials include pretests and posttests and begin with geometric shapes and move through passage reading.

The student who is changing to braille as a primary reading medium will probably be taken out of regular classroom for special one-to-one instruction in the code at a suitable time during the daily schedule. However, it is very important that the special teacher and the classroom teacher work together closely to strengthen the instruction, to provide positive motivation, and to integrate the student into classroom learning activities with sighted children as soon as possible. Frequently, the integration takes place first in the area of braille writing. When students first learn the formation of the braille alphabet letters necessary for spelling words, they begin by writing them only in full spelling. Later they write the words with contracted form as they learn the symbols for the contractions.

One way for the teacher to avoid assignments that result in slow, laborious reading is for the instructor to read orally as the student follows tactually. Of course, the teacher must pace the reading at a rate which challenges the student to move quickly, without losing the place. Periodically, the teacher may pause and allow the student to supply the next word or phrase.

A small percentage of blind adults learn to read braille with any degree of proficiency. The use of tape recordings and sighted readers makes listening a much easier and faster mode of gaining information from books. However, most blind adolescents and adults can master enough braille for use as a daily living skill. For example, many adults wish to learn enough to identify clothing, to write out and read receipes or telephone numbers, and to play cards games. To read braille well enough to enjoy books and periodicals is easier for the younger and more highly motivated pupils.

Motivation, age, finger sensitivity, attitude toward braille, intelligence, and need are all factors which should be considered in making a decision regarding braille emphasis. Special learning occurs in association with other disabilities such as cerebral palsy, deafness, mental retardation, diabetes, and heart trouble. For example, diabetics may have extreme difficulty at times in identifying braille characters. In some instances, it may be helpful to use a jumbo or enlarged braille (See Figure 35). Jumbo braille writers and slates can be obtained from the American Printing House for the Blind.

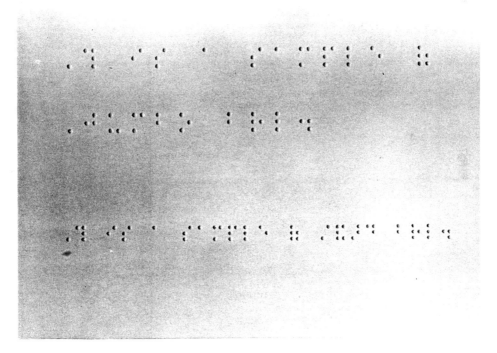

Figure 35. A comparison of jumbo and standard braille.

In the past, blind children and adults have been taught to read braille starting with Grade 1 and proceeding to Grade 1 1/2 and then to Grade 2. The Braille Series (Illinois Braille Committee of 1960, 1983) which has been popularly used with adults, uses this procedure. The advantages of this method are as follows:

1. It is easy for adults who want to start with a system (Grade 1) which is comparable to print reading.

2. Many adults may only be motivated to learn just enough braille to read simple labels, play cards, identify clothing, or write out and read recipes and telephone numbers.

Some teachers of the adult blind have objected to this technique because of the unlearning that must take place for those students who progress to Grade 2 braille. They point out that many of the words which were spelled out in Grade 1 braille of Volume I must later be contracted in Volumes II and III. The stilted language of the Grade 1, 1 1/2, and 2 exercises which are designed to provide practice on the newly introduced letters and signs is also an objectionable feature to some teachers who prefer materials which are of more interest to the students.

Weiss (1980) suggested that the newly blinded adult is helped by using guidelines (a series of braille X's) with double spacing between words and between lines of braille. The beginning exercises of the Illinois Braille Series utilize guidelines and extra space between lines with an enlarged cell which makes braille reading easier for tactually impaired adults. Later the spaces between the lines and the cells become smaller as the reader progresses through the lessons.

Jumbo-sized braille reading exercises for beginning late-blinded readers are provided in *Beginning Braille* by M. J. Tobin (Weiss, 1980). These exercises are supplemented by oral instruction on cassettes. Jumbo braille was successfully used with blind diabetic adults with decreased tactile sensitivity. These adults learned to use braille in daily living skills, such as reading clock faces, elevator buttons, telephone numbers, braille labels on clothes and food items. It was concluded that, although all blind diabetics may not need to learn to read braille, many could benefit from this training which could help make them more independent and employable. Clinical results from a study by Henrichs and Moorhouse (1969) indicated that the mean 2-point threshold in the diabetic subjects was 2.5 mm (as compared to 1.6 mm in the blind non-diabetic subjects). Since the distance between dots in standard braille is 2.2 mm, it was concluded that "difficulty" of the diabetic subjects in reading braille is probably related to the inability to perceive the individual points clearly.

"Jumbo" braille utilizes an enlarged braille cell with greater distances between dots. Two types of jumbo braille writers are produced by Howe Press of the Perkins School for the Blind. One uses enlarged dots within an enlarged cell and the other uses standard (sharp) dots with an enlarged cell. The latter arrangement would give more distance between the dots and is preferred by some users. Jumbo braille equipment and books can be obtained from three major sources of education materials for the blind and visually impaired: (1) Howe Press, (2) the American Printing House for the Blind, and (3) the Library of Congress. However, the number of books circulated by the Library of Congress is quite limited. Jumbo braille is really only practical at the present time as a source for beginners in braille who need an enlarged cell and for usage in daily living skills. Harley, Pichert, and Morrison (1986) found that through the use of jumbo braille tactually impaired blind diabetic adults could learn to read well enough for use in daily living skills, such as to read labels and telephone numbers.

Motivation for braille reading is extremely important for a successful program. If the blind person has a desire to learn braille for daily living needs, for job requirements, or for recreational purposes, it will be much easier. Some teachers start with card games for motivational purposes. Others use simple stories about subjects of interest to the reader. Craig (1975) used the following procedure:

1. Phase I: Short Episodes
    a. Simple stories are brailled episodes of related information on subjects of interest to the reader.
    b. Short sentences are double-spaced on separate lines, and words are double-spaced within a line.
    c. Vocabulary is limted, age-appropriate, simple, and repetitive.
    d. Grade 2 braille is used and movement along lines is emphasized.
    e. A whole word approach with emphasis on use of context cues is used.
    f. Use of ring and middle fingers is encouraged.
2. Phase II: Familiar Material
    a. Familiar songs and poetry are used.
    b. Punctuation and normal spacing are introduced.
    c. Students follow pages as the teacher reads.
    d. Contractions are not systematically developed.
3. Phase III: First Books
    a. Children's books are selected for adult interest and brailled.
    b. Single line spacing is used.
    c. Quotation marks and italics are introduced.
    d. Return sweeps are practiced.
4. Phase IV: First Press-Printed Books
    a. High interest low vocabulary books in braille are selected.
    b. Students continue to follow as the teacher reads.

5. Phase V: Silent Reading for Comprehension
   a. Silent reading is introduced.
   b. Comprehension is stressed through the use of meaningful material.
   c. Oral verbal paraphrasing is encouraged.
   d. Students tell each other the main points and question each other about the passages.
   e. Speed is developed through the key word approach. (Key words are identified on a quick first reading and re-reading is used to fill in details.)
   f. Drill on groups of words and sentences is emphasized rather than drill on single configurations.
   g. Braille writing is delayed until success in reading occurs.

The chief advantage of the Craig method is the emphasis on motivational materials which are presented in Grade 2 braille. However, it should be recognized that the program is designed for the more able and mature blind youths or adults. For those blind persons who do not need or desire to read braille books extensively, a Grade 1 program designed for use in daily living skills would be more practical.

The Language Master, a teaching machine using cards with a strip of recorded tape attached has been successful in teaching braille to blind adults (Weiss, 1980; Harley, Pichert & Morrison, 1986). Cards containing brailled letters and words have the letters and the words recorded on the strip of tape and give immediate feedback to the beginning braille reader. The machine permits the student to verify the letters without the aid of an instructor. After a few letters are learned tactually, the student can learn to write them with a braille writer or with a slate and stylus to reinforce the reading skill. A swing cell can be used to help the student learn the relative position of the dots in the cell in relation to the keys on the braille writer. Three holes in each of two rectangular blocks represent the spaces for the dots in a braille cell. Pegs are used in the holes to represent braille dots. In the vertical position the blocks represent the braille cell, in the horizontal position they represent the keys on the braille writer.

Relevant Braille is a correspondence course offered by the Hadley School for the Blind (Weiss, 1980). This course uses cassette instructions to teach the braille alphabet and numbers, and reading is reinforced by writing on a slate and stylus which is furnished to the student. Alternative systems to braille which are used mostly by adults in the United

Kingdom and the United States are Moon Print and the Fishburne Alphabet. The Moon embossed reading system was developed in 1847 by Dr. William Moon (Best, 1919). This system of embossed lines and dots, published by the Royal National Institute for the Blind in England and has been used on a small scale in America since 1870, has been more popular with the older visually impaired population. The Fishburne Alphabet for the Blind was designed for use by older blind adults who do not use braille for recording phone number, addresses, and labels. This system of embossed dots and lines has been reported to be easier to learn than braille dots (Newman & Hall, 1986).

SUMMARY

A most important factor in the braille reading program for the late newly blinded is the provision for success in reading since newly blinded persons are generally insecure and are very sensitive to failure. The attitude and skill of the remedial teacher are important factors to consider. If the teacher is well qualified in teaching braille, and high expectations are held for the pupils, good results can often be obtained. The teacher should carefully consider the reading needs of the pupil for braille reading and his reading potential based on a thorough assessment of his abilities. The emotional, perceptual, and academic readiness of the person should be considered in planning a successful readiness program. After setting objectives for the reading program, the teacher should plan systematic activities to insure success from the very beginning. Lessons should be designed in small sequential steps, but the material should be interesting to the reader. Positive reinforcement should be given as much as possible in a way that encourages self-confidence. Successful learning experiences throughout the rehabilitation program should enable the newly blinded person to develop a positive self-concept and an adjustment to blindness which is conducive to good mental health.

CHAPTER 11

USE OF TECHNOLOGY IN TEACHING COMMUNICATION SKILLS

L ISTENING, speaking, reading, and writing have been discussed previously as four important facets of the child's communication system. Listening and speaking develop at an earlier age and provide the basis for the development of the latter two skills. When the child enters school, reading and writing become important methods of communication. Visually impaired and blind students are often excluded from reading and writing unless special provisions or adaptations are made in their materials. "If it were not for the partial solutions offered by reading braille, by reading print that is optically, electronically, or physically enlarged, and by reading by listening, blind and visually impaired persons would have to live under a severe handicap" (Foulke, 1981, p. 101).

TECHNOLOGY IN COMMUNICATION

Advances in technology have made many devices for visually impaired and blind persons which help to reduce their handicaps in the area of communication. These devices make information available in three ways: visually, auditorially, and tactually. These developments have improved the outlook for the visually impaired and will lead to greater independence for them. Teachers of visually impaired students should be aware of the expense involved with technology and the rapid changes that occur within industry. This chapter does not include descriptions of all technology available to the visually impaired, but provides an overview of most of the current technology. The reader is encouraged to seek other resources for more information. A list of resources is included in Appendix G. Microcomputers, one of the latest advancements in technology, are becoming valuable educational tools for visually impaired students and will be discussed separately.

Visual Access Devices

Pioneering efforts by Barraga (1964) and others have led to a greater number of visually impaired students using their remaining vision in greater degrees and more efficiently. Optical aids and electronic devices are being used more with the visually impaired in an effort to provide access to print materials.

Closed-Circuit Televisions. The closed-circuit television (CCTV) is an electronic optical aid which provides visually impaired students direct access to all printed material by enlarging the size of the print on a television monitor. The CCTV system consists of three major parts: (1) a monitor; (2) a small television camera with a variable zoom lens; and (3) a sliding reading stand on which to place the material to be read or written.

Brand (1976) described the use of the CCTV as an aid in the administration of psychological tests to partially sighted students. It was found that students perform significantly better when the CCTV was used in assessment. Rossi (1980) reported that in a study of the use of the CCTV in reading, seven of 10 students read faster within one month while using the CCTV. In addition to reading faster, Rossi reported that students could write on lined paper using regular pens and pencils and could stay within the lines while using the CCTV where they previously were unable to write letters smaller than an inch in size.

Israel (1973) described criteria for selecting a CCTV for purchase. He suggested that the individual should consider the following: magnification, focus, reversed image, sharpness, clarity, movable viewing table, adjustable monitor, portability, accessories, monitor selections, warranty and service, long-term support, and user's manual and instructions (p. 102).

The two major advantages of a a CCTV are the immediate accessibility of all printed materials (books, dittos, magazines, etc.) and the adaptability for writing activitites. CCTVs can also be used with typewriters so visually impaired typists can see their mistakes; they have high magnification, adjustable contrast, and they can greatly increase reading distance. Excessive cost (approximately $2,500) and the lack of portability are the two major disadvantages of the CCTV. The lack of portability is not as great a disadvantage for elementary students since they often stay in one room for the greater part of their day. The CCTV must usually be placed in a central location for junior high and high school students because of this lack of portability. Additional disadvantages include eye and muscle fatigue and the need for motor coordination on the part of the student in order to control the movement of the stand on which the reading material is placed.

Overhead Projectors. The over-head projector can be used with some visually impaired students during their classroom instruction. Bruce (1973) described the use of the overhead projector for instructing visually impaired and blind students in mathematics. Bruce suggested that the room be darkened by turning off the lights and closing the shades. Students should be allowed to move as close to the screen as needed. Bold line washable felt-tip pens and grease pencils work best on the clear plastic film. Colored markers can also be very effective in demonstrating concepts and important points. The teacher should describe each step orally so that blind students can benefit from the activity. Blind students should make notes in braille as information is dictated.

Bruce (1973) listed the following advantages to be gained through the use of the overhead projector:

1. The teacher can make use of educational materials to meet the needs of the students.
2. The attention of the students is focused at one location.
3. The lens can be focused to accommodate individual differences in vision.
4. The teacher is able to use his/her own demonstrations and descriptions.
5. Simultaneous use of auditory and visual input improves retention of material taught.

Overhead projectors can be a problem for some students in mainstreamed settings. Some students are unable to view the materials presented on an overhead projector at any distance. Adaptations should be made by providing visually impaired students with copies of the material presented on the overhead if possible. Classroom teachers should be made aware of the need to verbalize all information presented on the overhead so that visually impaired students who cannot see the screen are able to get the information.

Projection Magnifiers. Some visually impaired students can benefit from the use of projection magnifiers such as the Optiscope and the IBM Microfilm Viewer as reading aids. These optical instruments project images on a polarizing screen. The major advantage for using a projection magnifier with visually impaired students is that the screen can be viewed from any distance. Disadvantages include: (1) poor contrast at times, partly due to the glass on the screen and/or the lighting in the room, (2) limited degree of magnification (about 2 times), (3) distortion of print at times, and (4) reduced field of vision (Harley & Lawrence, 1984).

Anderson (1980) described a study conducted by the National Center for the Education of the Blind using microfiche as a reading aid for visually impaired students. The results showed that the microfiche is a valuable aid for reading. There are a number of disadvantages in using the microfiche as a reading aid with the visually impaired: (1) excessive cost of the microfiche equipment, (2) lack of availability of printed material, (3) equipment is not portable, and (4) inability to underline or make notes on the page. Generally the microfiche has not met early expectations.

Optical Aids. Optical aids are becoming more sophisticated and of higher quality. Students are relying on them more and more as a tool to gain access to printed material. There are two general categories of optical aids: near aids which allow the user to see at close distances and distance aids which allow the user to see at varying distances. Bradfield (1984) listed four types of near aids: (1) head-borne magnifiers, (2) stand magnifiers, (3) hand-held magnifiers, and (4) electronic magnifiers (The CCTV and Viewscan are discussed separately). Telescopes are optical aids for distance use. Telescopes can be used to read from the chalkboard in the classroom and to read street signs and markers while traveling. Optical aids are portable, relatively inexpensive, and they provide the student with easy access to most printed material. The major disadvantages are their restriction of the field of vision and eye fatigue from extended use.

Electronic Magnifier. The Viewscan (Wormald, Inc.) is an electronic magnifier that enlarges print and projects it on a screen. It consists of a miniature hand-scanned camera for reading printed text and a display screen capable of presenting images of characters up to 75-80 mm (3 inches) in height. (Viewscan also has an accompanying keyboard system called the Viewscan Text System which will be discussed later in the microcomputer section of this chapter.) The major advantage is the accessibility of all printed material. The major disadvantages are: (1) excessive cost, (2) the limited number of characters that appear on the screen at a time, and (3) students must have good motor coordination in order to move the camera across lines of print. However, Wormald reports reading speeds up to 300 wpm in an advertisement brochure.

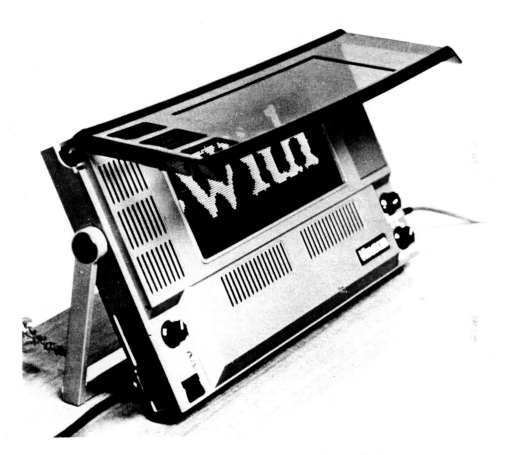

Figure 36. The Viewscan. Courtesy of Wormald, Inc.

Auditory Access Devices

A number of technological developments have been made in auditory access devices in recent years. Examples of some of these devices will be briefly described below. A more thorough discussion of relevant research and techniques for teaching listening skills are provided in this book in the chapter on listening.

Talking Books. The Library of Congress began distributing talking books to the blind in 1934. Specially designed record players, called talking-book machines, were developed at the American Foundation for the Blind. They play records which are recorded at slower than conventional speeds and are produced by the National Library Service for the Blind and Physically Handicapped of the Library of Congress. The records and talking book machines are distributed free of charge to visually impaired individuals through a nationwide network of cooperating libraries. Catalogs listing books (records, cassette tapes, large print, and braille) are available from the Regional Libraries for the Blind and Physically Handicapped. Textbooks and instructional materials are not available on talking book. Supplemental instructional talking books can be purchased from the American Printing House for the Blind in Louisville, Kentucky.

Tape Players. The Library of Congress also provides specially designed cassette tape players and cassettes, which are recorded at slower than conventional speeds. The slower speed and the use of four tracks instead of the standard two tracks allows more material to be recorded per cassette. The slow speed prevents the tape from being used in a conventional tape recorder and protects the copyright of the publisher who has made a special waiver for use with visually impaired persons. Tape players and cassette tapes are loaned free to visually impaired persons qualifying for the service. The American Printing House for the Blind has done extensive work designing tape recorders with variable speed controls and the capacity to index material. Tape players and supplemental instructional cassette tapes from the American Printing House may be purchased through the quota system. Recordings for the Blind provides textbooks to school-age visually impaired persons free of charge. Cassette tape recorders are generally more popular than talking book machines because of their portability, ease of use, and greater variety of taped materials.

Compressed speech and accelerated speech are two techniques that are helpful in providing visually impaired students quantities of information in a shorter period of time. Although originally, mechanical devices were used to delete segments of the speech signal to accomplish compressed speech, computers are now used. Natural pauses occurring in speech are shortened or eliminated in the production of some compressed speech. Speech synthesis is another method for compressing speech. Accelerated speech is speech that is played on a tape player at a faster than normal rate. This method is often described as having the Donald Duck effect because the pitch and intelligibility are changed. The American Printing House for the Blind specially adapts tape players so that listeners can control the speed at which they play cassette tapes (Bischoff, 1979).

Synthetic Speech Devices. The Kurzweil Reading Machine (KRM) is an example of an electronic speech output reading aid. It consists of a clear glass top on which a printed page is placed face-down above an optical scanner, a control panel, a computer and a voice output device. The greatest advantages of the KRM are: (1) direct access to printed materials, (2) the relatively little training required for use, (3) controls which allow for high reading speeds (Goodrich, Bennett, De L'aune, Lauer & Mowinski, 1979). The major disadvantages include the excessive cost of the machine, the frequent need for costly maintenance, and the lack of portability.

Other Talking Aids. A variety of other aids have been adapted with speech output and are invaluable to the visually impaired. Although these aids are not used during direct instruction in comunication skills, some examples are worth noting. Examples include: talking calculators, talking telephone directories, clocks, bathroom scales, and blood pressure kits.

Tactual Access Devices

Blind students generally use two types of tactual materials; they read braille or they read print using the Optacon. Reading rates using both methods are slower than normally sighted reading rates and require extensive training in order to obtain proficiency. Blind students may learn to emboss braille but the Optacon is a technology developed for reading only.

Manual Braille Writers. The Perkins Brailler is an all-purpose writing aid for blind students. It is available from Howe Press and can be purchased on quota from the American Printing House for the Blind. It has a unimanual conversion that can be used with individuals who must use only one hand and enlarged braille cells can be produced by braille machines which have been adapted for tactually impaired blind adults. The Cranmer Modified Perkins Brailler, a computer terminal/printer based on the Perkins Brailler, will be discussed in the section on microcomputers.

The Lavender Brailler, although no longer on the market, is still available in some state material centers and residential schools. It is a writing aid similar to the Perkins Brailler. The outer case is made of plastic and is more compact and lighter weight than the Perkins Brailler. It is not as mechanically dependable as the Perkins Brailler.

The slate and stylus is used by blind persons to take notes. It is small, compact, portable, inexpensive, and quieter than the brailler. Users must have good hand and finger control in order to manipulate the slate and stylus. Users must also have a good command of the braille code before they can write on the slate and stylus, as they must write letters and words backwards — from right to left.

Electronic Braille Writers. Technologists have developed a number of braille reading, writing, and audio tape recording machines that promise to be valuable tools in the education, careers, and leisure activities of blind people. The first of these machines was the Digicassette, which was developed in France. The Braillex was developed in Germany, and the VersaBraille and Microbrailler was developed in The United States (Mellor, 1979).

Electronic braille machines, also referred to as paperless braille machines, employ sophisticated microprocessors which enable them to store and retrieve information written on the braille keyboard. Braille characters are displayed via pins protruding through holes in the display panel on top of the machine. One line of braille characters is presented at a time. When the student has read the displayed braille, a button is pushed which causes a new line of braille to appear. Words that will not fit at the end of the display are automatically carried over to the following line.

Electronic braille machines have a braille keyboard which is composed of a key for each of the six braille dots and a key for spacing. The keys are used to braille information which is entered by a special code onto a cassette tape or a computer disk. These machines also have additional operational keys which allow the user to search for and retrieve information with relative ease.

Electronic braille machines have a wide variety of uses. They can be used as notetaking devices in the classroom. Word processing is probably the most important use of these machines, especially with their capacity to be interfaced with electric typewriters and printers. As specially recorded tapes and disks become more available, students will be able to read their textbooks and other materials using electronic braille machines. These machines are also used for data processing and as computer terminals.

There are a number of advantages for using electronic braille writers. These devices are portable and easy to operate. The tapes and disks used with these machines take up much less space than braille books and the tapes/disks are easier to produce and distribute than braille books. The cost of preparing tapes and disks on electronic braille machines will be much less than the cost of preparing regular braille books. These devices are quieter and more convenient than standard braillers.

Excessive cost and maintenance are probably the major disadvantages of electronic braille machines. These machines are not suitable for tables, graphs, or complex mathematical equations because only one line of braille can be displayed at a time. Finally, students need relatively good hand coordination and intelligence in order to read, write, and control the operational functions of these machines.

Optacon. The Optacon can be a valuable tool for the visually impaired student because it provides independent access to printed materials. The Optacon converts print into tactile images of the letters through the use of a small hand-held camera and a set of 144 vibrating pins. The camera is moved across a line of print and signals are sent from the camera to a tactile array which simultaneously provides enlarged reproductions of whatever the camera "sees" using the raised, vibrating pins. The user reads by placing the index finger of one hand on the tactile display while moving the camera across a line of print with the other hand (Goldish & Taylor, 1974).

The major advantages of an Optacon are its portability and the provision of independent access to printed materials. Major disadvantages include: (1) excessive cost, (2) costly maintenance, (3) slow reading speed, (4) the need for good motor coordination in order to move the camera along lines of print, and (5) the need for extensive training to learn to recognize the shapes of letters and numbers.

Microcomputers and the Visually Impaired

During the past few decades advances in technology have made a significant impact on the lives of visually impaired people, especially in their education, rehabilitation, and employment. Dupress (1963) stated that two of the most critical needs of visually impaired persons are the optimum use of their remaining senses and access to printed material. Microcomputers and the access technology to them may prove to be the single most promising effort yet for meeting these needs.

Most of the developments that have made computers and microcomputers accessible to the visually impaired have been developed in the past 10 years. In an early attempt to develop computer-assisted instruction in mathematics and reading for hearing impaired and visually impaired students, the Cincinnati public schools found that access technology for the visually impaired was not available (Morgan, 1975).

In one of the first studies documenting the use of computers with visually impaired students, Evans and Simpkins (1972) described a computer-assisted math program at Overbrook School for the Blind in which 43 children in fourth, fifth, and sixth grades used computers in their math classes. Three typewriter-like keyboard terminals were connected by a telephone in the classroom to a Hewlett-Packard computer housed at another location. A braille adaptor, manufactured by Triformation Systems, Inc. was used to print braille characters on a kind of ticker tape. The students in the study worked at a terminal on a rotating schedule for 20 minutes each day. The computer automatically signed the students off at the end of the allotted time. The computer was programmed to allow the students to try to answer a problem three times before it provided the correct response. At the end of each lesson, the student was told the total number of correct and incorrect responses. The computer automatically advanced the students to the next level when they achieved a certain percentage. Otherwise, the students repeated the lesson as needed. Although no data were provided regarding student progress, the article provided valuable descriptions of technical problems encountered in the study.

Instruction regarding the use of computers and microcomputers is often more complicated and involved for visually impaired students. While sighted students and students with some visual limitations are taught to operate microcomputers, severely visually impaired students must also learn how to use the access technology and how to use the microcomputer and the access technology together. Ryan and Bedi (1978) described a computer literacy course taught as early as 1977 at Bernard M. Baruch College, the City University of New York (CUNY). Fifteen visually impaired students were provided with knowledge and skills in computer technology for the visually impaired. A Triformation LED 120 high speed braille terminal was connected to the main computer at CUNY and used for the course. Partially sighted students also used Visualtek closed circuit televisions which enlarged print and displayed the image on a T.V. monitor. Although no data were provided, the workshop was reported a success.

Brunken (1984) described the use of technology at the Nebraska School for the Visually Handicapped (NSVH). Students received training on the Apple microcomputer and the various access components (Optacon, VersaBraille, etc.) utilizing materials designed by Brunken and training modules developed at Peabody College of Vanderbilt University. Brunken listed eight levels of utilization of microcomputers by the students and teachers at NSVH: tutorial, computer literacy, prevocational, personal-use application, programming, career planning, word processing, and administrative.

Sanford (1984) described a study of the use of an instructional program designed to teach visually impaired students to use microcomputers which was developed at Peabody College of Vanderbilt University. Results of the study indicated that braille students ages 12 years to 18 years and with IQs ranging from 84 to 120 were able to complete the instructional modules which taught the use of the Apple microcomputer and the access devices in the relatively short period of time. Results also showed, although not statistically significant for either group, that there was an overall increase in both students' and teachers' positive attitudes toward microcomputers during the study.

Koenig, Mack, Schenk, & Ashcroft (1985) reported on a study currently being conducted at the Tennessee School for the Blind in Nashville, Tennessee. Peabody College and the Tennessee School for the Blind were jointly awarded a 2-year grant from the Apple Education Foundation for the purpose of studying the development of word processing skills by visually impaired students. The study had two major goals: (1) the teachers were expected to become proficient users of microcomputers, the access technology, and the Braille-Edit (word processing) program, and (2) the visually impaired students were expected to develop writing and word processing skills. The major focus was to determine if braille word processing would allow blind students the freedom to write and make corrections more easily.

Uses of Microcomputers

Microcomputers may be used instructionally with visually impaired students in a number of ways: (1) computer-assisted instruction (CAI), also called computer-based instruction (CBI), (2) computer-managed instruction, and (3) word processing. Computer-assisted instruction is a method in which a computer is used to present instructional material to a learner. Specific modes of presentation of CAI materials to students include: (1) drill-and-practice, (b) tutorial, (c) simulation, (d) games, and (e) problem solving. In contrast, CMI is defined as an instructional management process, including perhaps CAI activities, as well as traditional forms of instruction. Computer-managed instruction has one or all of the following characteristics: (a) organizing curricula and student data, (b) monitoring student progress, (c) diagnosing and prescribing, (d) evaluating learning outcomes, and (e) providing planning for teachers. Microcomputers are also used for word processing, assessment and evaluation of students, and programming.

Drill and Practice. The drill and practice mode is used to drill students on information and material that has been previously introduced and or learned. It is used to supplement other forms of instruction (Budoff & Hutten, 1982). Drill and practice programs allow students to progress at their own rate, and provide instant feedback, and a variety of reinforcement. The computer is able to monitor very complex drill-and-practice activities which can be individualized to each student's needs (Foreman, 1983).

Tutorial. Tutorial programs present information or material to students for the first time, usually in a programmed format. The computer acts as a "tutor" for the student and teaches information, skills, and concepts. Tutorial programs can be written so that a student may remediate, review, or move ahead as needed.

Simulation. Software can be designed to simulate or generate real situations in the environments so the learner can manipulate variables and explore situations without having to experience the situations in real life. Oftentimes, the "controllable worlds" are too expensive, too dangerous, or just impossible to explore in real life (Foreman, 1983). Although these activities are designed to simulate some reality, game features can be incorporated into the programs to increase interest and learning (Budoff & Hutten, 1982).

Games. Computer games can be a very motivating and interesting way to help students develop problem-solving methods and strategies. A number of studies have been conducted to determine the motivational aspects of games (Malone, 1981; Frederiksen, Warren, Gillote, & Weaver, 1982; and Chaffin, Maxwell, & Thompson, 1982). Important motivational features of games include: immediate feedback, different levels of challenge, clear goals, fast pace, potential for improvement through familiarity and strategy, unlimited ceiling of performance, and possibly graphics, sound and color. Games can be developed to teach and provide a wide variety of subject matter, especially if the motivational considerations are incorporated.

Programming. Learning to program a computer is one of the best ways to teach problem solving because students must utilize all of the steps involved in the problem-solving method. Papert, a mathematician at Massachusetts Institute of Technology, developed a programming language which is simple enough for children to use. Young children are able to use such software as Papert's LOGO to learn how to program (Miller, 1983). LOGO may be especially useful with handicapped children because they are able to make decisions and see the consequences of their decisions immediately on the computer.

Word Processing. Word processing has the potential for increasing the quality, quantity, and creativity in students' writing assignments. Students are able to write information using the microcomputer without the constraints of proper spelling, grammar, and formating because corrections and changes are easily made. After the teacher grades a written assignment, marks errors, and makes suggestions for improvement, the student is able to make the corrections without having to retype the complete paper. Word processing promotes proofreading because it is easier to make corrections. Students can be more creative because it is easier to add and delete information. With the appropriate access equipment, students are able to produce a print and braille copy of their work and produce a "perfect" paper with no braille erasures (Brunken, 1984).

Data Management. Microcomputers can help teachers and administrators manage paperwork. Microcomputers are being used in school business management, budgeting, purchasing, inventories, attendance, and personnel management. The continual growth of federal and state regulations cause a need for educational management systems at each level of education (school, county, state, federal). Microcomputers can be an excellent tool for processing information and reporting required data to the government, to parents, and to others (Joiner, Sedlak, Silverstein, & Densel, 1980).

Microcomputers can serve as a data management and retrieval system for IEPs, objectives, assessment scores, and student records. In short, the microcomputer can serve as a tireless teacher's aid. The microcomputer can assist the teacher with repetitious paper and pencil work and in recording and plotting data. Stored data can be easily transformed into charts or displayed graphically, which will provide the student and the teacher information about the student's progress (Ashcroft & Young, 1981).

Diagnostics and Assessment. Microcomputers are being used increasingly to assist teachers in diagnosing and assessing student performance. The microcomputer has been found to be fast, reliable, and more accurate than human examiners.

There are a number of other advantages for using the computer to diagnose student performance. Microcomputers allow frequent evaluation which could lead to increased pupil achievement. Okey (1976) stated that frequent diagnostic testing of students leads to higher pupil achievement. Microcomputers are not time conscious; they do not rush the student (unless they are programmed to do so). They also eliminate the need for stop watches. They are non-threatening to the student, remove biases of the examiner, and have extensive recordkeeping capacity and analytic power.

Advantages of Microcomputers with Visually Impaired Students

Microcomputers are demonstrating their potential for enhancing the lives of visually impaired people. Although new hardware and software are being developed daily, microcomputers currently offer unique advantages to the visually impaired.

Flexibility. Microcomputers are designed so they are flexible enough to be used by both normal and handicapped students. Students in the same class can complete lessons at different levels using the microcomputer, although some visually impaired students may require equipment that make the microcomputer accessible.

User Friendly. Microcomputers can be programmed to be "user friendly." They can use the student's name in the lessons, and provide positive feedback to the child in a non-threatening and non-judgemental manner. They can be programmed to provide step-by-step directions and lead the student through an activity to insure mastery of skills with little failure.

Instant Feedback. Microcomputers can be programmed to provide instant feedback, thus alleviating some of the stress associated with waiting for feedback to responses. The immediacy of the feedback is reinforcing to the students since they do not have to wait for the teacher to grade their work.

Self-Paced. Students are able to progress at their own rates when they use microcomputers. Visually impaired students often work at a slower pace than normal students. The microcomputer can be programmed to wait for a response (Shiffman, Tobin, & Buchanan, 1982). The student can move as rapidly or as slowly as needed and can review material at any time (Hannaford, 1983). Teachers of visually impaired students should carefully select software that has been programmed to include a selection for speed of response or that is slow enough for their students to complete the activities without becoming frustrated. Drill and practice activities can be programmed to include a timer. Students are able to increase their speed of certain skills by competing against the timer and their previous scores.

Multisensory. Microcomputers can provide a multisensory approach to learning (Hannaford & Sloan, 1981). Access equipment and software have been developed which provide multisensory instruction via tactual display, sound, text, graphics, and animation. Hannaford (1983) stated that handicapped students often function much better when the material is presented through a multisensory approach. Perhaps most important is the ability to make drill-and-practice activities more interesting by adding sound effects, animation, and game playing situations (Budoff & Hutten, 1982; Schiffman, Tobin, & Buchanan, 1982). The use of multisensory instruction, especially animation, graphics, and game activities will present a problem for severely visually impaired students, because the access equipment used by these students currently do not function with programs that include these characteristics.

Disadvantages of Microcomputers with Visually Impaired

Although microcomputers can aid instruction and benefit handicapped students, both teachers of the visually impaired and their students need to be aware of certain disadvantages and problems. Following is a brief description of some of the major disadvantages of using micrcomputers with visually impaired students.

Interfacing Hardware. Probably the greatest problem for teachers and students is interfacing microcomputers with the access equipment and keeping them working together. Teachers are often intimidated by technical information presented in accompanying manuals and shy away from handling problems as they occur with the equipment. Often the information is so technical or complex that lay persons are unable to understand and translate enough to follow the directions. There is a great need for schools to purchase service contracts for their microcomputers and the access equipment so they can be maintained in working condition. It is also essential to identify a person with technical skills to call as problems arise.

Using Software. The nature of the needs of visually impaired students has caused the development of special software to help mitigate those needs. For example, software has been developed that provides speech output and large print on the microcomputer. Teachers and students sometimes find it difficult to boot and run such programs. If the exact sequence of commands are not used properly, the program will not run. This can be very frustrating. In addition, back-up copies of software should be purchased or made so that if programs are destroyed or damaged, the student will still have access to the program via the back-up copy.

Expensive. Microcomputers are becoming more affordable, but they are still too expensive for students to have easy access to them in the classrooms. Many school systems are making it a top priority to have at least one microcomputer in each school. Even so, there are not sufficient numbers of microcomputers available for regular or special education students. In addition, although microcomputers are becoming less expensive and more available, the equipment that makes microcomputers accessible to visually impaired students is very expensive. Some of the access equipment costs more than the microcomputer to which it is connected.

Software can also be very expensive. Educators should become knowledgeable of various resources, such as Minnesota Educational Computer Consortium (MECC), which provide software to educational agencies at reduced prices or group rates. There is also an abundance of software that is considered public domain and can be easily copied with little or no cost except for the price of a blank disk. Finding appropriate software to use with visually impaired students can be difficult. There is a need for a clearinghouse for software that can be used with visually impaired students; the software may need to be grouped by their compatibility with various pieces of access technology.

Accessibility. Microcomputers present information visually on a monitor and require typed responses on a keyboard which makes it impossible for some visually impaired students to use them. Technology is currently available and is continually being developed and improved that provide access to microcomputers for visually impaired students. Goodrich (1984) stated that the rapidly changing nature of the computer industry is a major concern for visually impaired persons because changes have the potential for denying access to microcomputers.

Reading Disability. Unless there has been a special adaptation made, such as accessing the microcomputer with a voice synthesizer, most information presented on the microcomputer is visual in nature.

Students with reading problems may experience difficulty in interacting with the microcomputer. In addition, many of the commercially-available programs are single spaced, which makes reading even more difficult for some students (Grimes, 1981). The same problem exists for students who read braille. Students who use the VersaBraille as an access tool, but have difficulty reading and writing braille will have problems interacting with the microcomputer.

Need for Typing Skills. The nature of the microcomputer requires that a student type a response in order to interact with a program. Although it is generally recommended that visually impaired students be taught typing at an earlier age than regular students, this recommendation is not always followed. Using the hunt-and-peck method slows down instruction time and is often an impossible task for very low vision students. Lack of typing skills is especially critical when a student is using the microcomputer as a word processor.

Fragmentation of Instruction and Curriculum. Currently most teachers do not have access to microcomputer programs that match perfectly with the curriculum in their classroom. It is difficult to maintain consistency and continuity of instruction when teachers do not have access to a wide variety of software to meet the instructional needs of their students. Teachers should preview software so they will not present material out of sequence.

Methods of Accessing Microcomputers

Students in programs for the visually impaired may have acuities ranging from 20/50 to no light perception, a limited field of vision, or both. Teachers of visually impaired students need to be aware of the wide range of visual functioning of their students. A large number of visually impaired students can use microcomputers without any special adaptations. They are able to read from the screen and use the keyboard to interact with the microcomputer just as normally seeing people do. However, there is a portion of the visually impaired population who, because of the degree of their visual loss, cannot read from a standard screen or have a meaningful interaction with a standard keyboard. A variety of devices have been developed which enable these visually impaired people to have access to microcomputers. Each type of access device and method will be discussed in the following sections.

Standard Screen and Keyboard. As mentioned in the previous paragraph, many visually impaired students are able to use microcomputers without any adaptations. These students are able to read from the standard-sized monitor, type on the keyboard, and read the print-outs which are normal print size. Teachers should be aware of the different print sizes which are generated by different microcomputers and by the same microcomputer when certain features are changed. For example, the print size on an Apple microcomputer is normally presented in 40 columns but when an 80 column card is added, the print size is reduced by half. It would be much easier for a visually impaired student to read the larger print presented in 40 columns than the smaller print produced by the 80 column card.

Contrast is another important consideration when assessing the needs of visually impaired students for using microcomputers. Students should be taught how to adjust the contrast on the microcomputer. Some teachers of visually impaired students have had success in increasing contrast by turning off the lights in a part of the room, closing window shades, or using a color monitor.

Teachers of visually impaired students may want to include a statement of how a student functions with the print on a microcomputer screen as part of their assessment of a student's functional vision. This author has been asked to include such a diagnosis and statement about students who were given assessments of their functional vision for staffing into the vision program; the classroom teachers planned to use microcomputers with the students for instruction and wanted to make sure the students could read the print on the screen.

Standard Screen with Selected Software. If a visually impaired student is unable to read the standard-sized print on the microcomputer screen, teachers should be aware that there is a wide range of educational software available with varying print size. A review of available software may reveal certain programs that have bold pictures and enlarged print. Some visually impaired students who cannot read regular print may have success in using such programs.

Teachers of visually impaired students should also identify available software that help to teach visual efficiency skills. Programs are becoming available that teach such skills as same and different, color discrimination, matching patterns, and various other visual perception skills. The microcomputer can be a very motivating tool to use in teaching these skills to visually impaired students.

Standard Screen with Optical Aids. About 80% of the people who are classified as legally blind retain some useful vision (Ruconich, 1984). Low-vision aids can be an inexpensive and effective means of gaining access to microcomputers. Goodrich (1984) stated that with the possible exception of replacing or originally purchasing a higher quality monitor, microcomputers do not require adaptations with low vision aids. Oftentimes, the standard monitor does not have clear, sharp print that is needed by a low vision student. Television monitors may also be purchased in many sizes; the larger screens can be helpful for the visually impaired student.

Visually impaired students use the same low-vision aids with the microcomputer as they use for near reading tasks. Examples include hand-held magnifiers, hand-borne magnifiers, and stand magnifiers. These aids have the same limitations with microcomputers as they do with other near-reading tasks, namely, limited size of field, the need for a constant focal distance, reduced illumination, the necessity of using a hand with the hand-held or stand magnifier (which hinders typing speed), and eye fatigue after prolonged use. The aids are inexpensive and provide total access to a microcomputer without any modifications (Goodrich, 1984). Teachers of visually impaired students may consider adjusting the placement of the monitor so that it is directly in front of the student's face. This placement may help to decrease posture fatigue, especially while using low vision aids.

Standard Screen with Closed-Circuit Television. The closed-circuit television is another example of a low-vision aid that can be used with the microcomputer to enlarge the print size for visually impaired students. Closed-circuit televisions are more expensive than the other low vision aids previously discussed, and the choice of using a CCTV over one of the other aids should be thoroughly assessed. CCTVs are appropriate for a smaller percentage of the visually impaired population than the other access methods discussed so far.

Enlarged Print Using Software. Large print can be generated on the microcomputer monitor by using specially designed software. Examples of such software programs are Braille Edit and the newer Braille Express by David Halliday. Braille Express has the capability of enlarging the print on the screen allowing students to complete word processing activities in large print. They are not able to use the disk to enlarge other programs; for example, they cannot load Braille Edit and then run another program in large print. Magic Slate is another word processing program that is capable of producing a variety of print sizes ranging from 20, 40, to 80 columns for the print. Twenty column print is twice as large as the standard 40 column print, and 80 column print is half as large as the 40 column print. A large number of visually impaired students would be able to read the print on the screen of the microcomputer and from print-outs while using the 20 column print produced by Magic Slate.

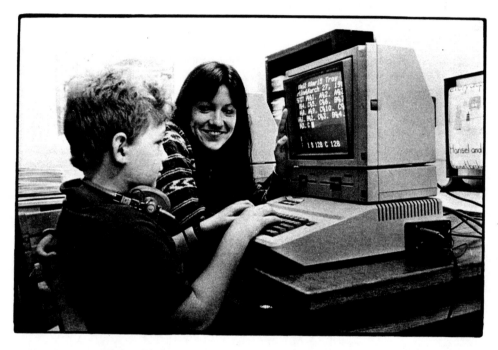

Figure 37. Enlarged print using software.

Speech Enterprises of Houston, Texas, is disseminating a disk that will enlarge the print size of some programs. The microcomputer is booted with the print enlarger disk, then the program to be enlarged is placed in the disk drive. The enlarger disk will only work with disks that can be booted by typing "catalog." The print size is large enough for low vision students to read and can be a good device for low vision students to use for writing microcomputer programs. A major advantage is the cost; it is relatively inexpensive compared to other access devices. There are a number of disadvantages: (1) 24 characters are scrolled up too quickly for some low vision students to read, (2) the enlarger program will not work with programs that have graphics, and (3) words are split at the end of lines which can cause additional problems for students who have reading difficulties (Schenk, 1985).

Teachers of visually impaired students should be aware that enlarged print can be used with a large portion of visually impaired students. Some students who read braille for all practical purposes may be able to read the enlarged print produced by specially designed software for word processing or programming activities. Compared to some of the other access devices, the use of software to enlarge the size of the print on the microcomputer screen is a relatively inexpensive method and should be used with students when appropriate.

Large-Print-Computers. A number of microcomputers have been designed expressly for the purpose of providing large print for partially sighted individuals. Large print computers provide variable-size letters and controls to maximize the contrast for the viewer. The material on the screen has sufficient magnification to be used by most students with some residual vision. In considering the purchase and use of large print microcomputers with visually impaired students, teachers should be aware that there is a great reduction in the amount of information displayed on the monitor. Students are able to view only a few words at a time. This limits the use and effectiveness of much of the software that is on the market. Goodrich (1984) pointed out that using the large print computer with certain programs can be very time consuming. He stated they are easiest to use for computer programming and with software that is line-oriented instead of screen-oriented.

Wormald produces a portable large print microcomputer called the Viewscan Text System. Students are able to use the portable microcomputer much the same as they would a regular microcomputer. The portable microcomputer has the capability of being interfaced with a variety of accessories, including a standard-size microcomputer, printer, telephone modem, and mainframe system. Again, teachers and students need to be aware of the restriction of the amount of material displayed on the screen at one time. The portable microcomputer can only display a few letters at a time which can be time consuming and bothersome during certain microcomputer activities.

Voice-Synthesizers. Voice synthesizers have become readily available and widely used. They are a very promising means of accessing microcomputers for the blind and visually impaired. Voice synthesis is analogous to printing the screen to voice. There are two methods of producing speech from the microcomputer. Digitized prerecorded speech is one method. The other method, and the more popular form, is synthetic speech in which electronically generated sounds are put together to form words. In general, voice synthesizers have the capability of pronouncing words, letters, punctuation, and some are able to review. Review features enable a person to scan a document or listen to certain sections again.

Synthetic speech terminals allow a significant increase in the rate in which blind and visually impaired persons can get information from a microcomputer. Generally students will need to become accustomed to the speech produced by the voice-synthesizer. Speeds of 360 to 400 words per minute have been reported. Goodrich (1984) stated that it is common for users to work at speeds of 200 words per minute which is much faster than large print and braille reading rates.

Electronic Braille. Electronic braille, also called refreshable braille or paperless braille, has the potential for being the most effective means of gaining access to microcomputers for proficient braille users (Goodrich, 1984). Electronic braillers can be used as stand alone devices, as previously discussed in this chapter, and as an access tool for the microcomputer. The braille student can use the electronic brailler to send and receive information from the microcomputer.

There are several advantages for utilizing electronic braille machines as access devices for microcomputers: (1) information can be more quickly read and produced than with the Optacon, (2) there is immediate feedback of information entered into the microcomputer, (3) the devices have extensive memory capacity, (4) the devices are relatively portable, and (5) the devices can be used as input and output devices (Goodrich, 1984; Ruconich, 1984). Disadvantages include: (1) excessive cost, (2) costly maintenance, (3) the search for particular information is more difficult and time consuming because only one line of information is presented at a time, (4) normal braille reading speeds are slowed down due to the difficulty in reading grades, 1, 2, and 3 braille, Nemeth Code, and computer braille, (5) reading speeds are also decreased because of the need to move the hands back and forth from the braille keyboard to the tactile display, (6) information stored on tapes and disks cannot be interchanged among the different brands of electronic devices and not all manufacturers use the same computer braille code, and (7) tactile graphics and tabular materials cannot be displayed appropriately for the reader (Goodrich, 1984; Ruconich, 1984).

Although commercial production is not yet possible, work is being done on the development of a full-page refreshable display which would solve some of the problems associated with the electronic braille machine. The full-page display would function similar to the electronic brailler, but instead of a single line of braille, 25 rows by 40 columns of braille would be displayed at a rapid rate. Major advantages would be the provision of larger blocks of information for the braille reader to read, scan, and edit and the provision of two-dimensional graphs and charts (Goodrich, 1984). Excessive cost and maintenance will most likely be the major disadvantages of such a device.

Paper Braille. Before the inventions of electronic braille machines, the major access to computers was through paper-braille printing devices such as the LED-120 printer from Triformation Systems, Inc. These high speed printers can produce braille from a keyboard, from a computer, from magnetic cassettes or from almost any source of coded information. When appropriate computer programs are used, these printers can produce graphics, maps, charts, bar graphs, and diagrams (Goodrich, 1984). The major advantage is the speed of grade 1 and grade 2 braille production. The major disadvantages of these nonportable paper printers are their price, costly maintenance, size, and noise.

The Cranmer Modified Perkins Brailler (CMPB), available from Triformation Systems in Stuart, Florida, allows students to send information to the computer via the braille keyboard and receive information from the computer via braille pages printed by the CMPB. The electronic modification is housed in a box attached to the bottom of the brailler. The CMPB can be linked to peripheral devices. The CMPB has a number of advantages: (1) it is much less expensive than other hardcopy printers such as the LED-120, (2) it provides a full-page display where electronic braillers cannot, (3) students have access to materials presented in columns which is not possible with electronic braillers, and (4) it can produce tactile graphics which greatly increased the variety of programs available to braille students (Ruconich, 1984).

A major limitation of the portable Cranmer Brailler is its slow printing (embossing) speed. The CMPB does not have continuous paper feed which makes it time-consuming because each sheet of paper must be inserted, monitored, and removed by hand. It is noisy, heavier than desirable, and the cassette tapes cannot be interchanged with other electronic braille devices, nor can it use tapes from other braille devices (Ruconich, 1984). Goodrich (1984) pointed out that mechanical unreliability is another problem with the CMPB. Goodrich (1984) stated that there are additional problems when using the hardcopy printed as a computer terminal: (1) slow printing speed, (2) lack of knowledge of the position of the cursor, (3) the need to move one's hand from the keyboard to the printed material and back limits reading speed, and (4) the proximity of the embossing head hinders reading.

Although the Cranmer Brailler was the first portable electronic paper braille printer on the market, new and improved paper printers such as the ones from VisualTeck and Howe Press are becoming available. Hopefully, some of the discussed problems will be mitigated with the development of newer models and products.

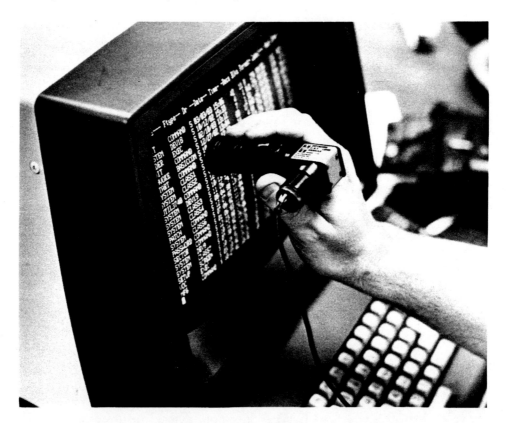

Figure 38. The Optacon can be used to gain access to information on the microcomputer screen.

Optacon. Ruconich (1984) stated that because of early availability, the Optacon was probably the most widely used computer access technology for tactual readers. Even so, it has the potential to serve the fewest users, especially with the advent of electronic braille machines. The reader uses a specially designed cathode ray tube lens which is attached to the Optacon camera to read the video display of the microcomputer. The regular camera lens of the Optacon is used to read paper print-outs. The ability to read both paper print-outs and from the video display is probably the primary advantage of the Optacon. The reader has immediate access to all information from the computer; material presented in columns and in graphic form can be easily scanned. Although students can read information using the Optacon, information cannot be sent to the microcomputer via the Optacon. They must use the microcomputer keyboard to enter information into the keyboard.

There are a number of disadvantages for using the Optacon as an access method. The major disadvantage is the training time necessary to become proficient in the use of the Optacon. Telesensory (1978) reported reading speeds from 20 to 60 words per minute using the Optacon. These speeds would most likely be even slower when reading from the video display of the microcomputer. Ruconich (1984) stated that students must have good bimanual coordination and learn to align the Optacon camera properly in order to read from the screen. Students may require additional training so they can read various print styles and learn to hold, align, and track using the special attachment on a vertical video screen. In addition, cost and maintenance are major limitations, as with almost all other access methods.

Considerations for Selecting Software

The microcomputer can be an invaluable teaching aid for visually impaired students with appropriate access and if appropriate educational programs or software are used. Careful consideration should be given to the selection of software that meets the needs of the learners and the needs of the teacher. There is an abundance of literature available regarding the evaluation and selection of educational software to meet the needs of students in regular education and in special education programs. "Software to be utilized with visually impaired students should meet the criteria which are relevant to the selection of quality software for any student and any educational application" (Ashcroft, 1984, p. 115).

Educational software should be evaluated regarding general considerations such as reliability, warranty, support from supplier, appropriateness of the documentation, and ease of use. Hannaford and Sloan (1981) developed an extensive list of systematic criteria that allows for appropriate selection of educational software for handicapped students.

The questionnaire is divided into three major areas of learner/teacher needs, instructional integrity, and technical adequacy and utility. Examples of specific considerations include: relevancy to instructional needs, format appeal, sequence of instruction, developmental steps, accurate and clear content, clear instructions, and ability to be used independently by students.

After the teacher of visually impaired students has evaluated educational software to determine the quality and appropriateness in general, additional concerns must be addressed which are relevant to the particular access mode being utilized. The teacher should try out the software with the particular piece(s) of access equipment that will be utilized with the students. Following are some specific considerations that must be utilized in the selection of software if visually impaired students are to use microcomputers effectively. Many of these considerations were identified as part of a federal grant at George Peabody College of Vanderbilt University (Ashcroft, 1984).

Regular Print Concerns. Is the print large enough and clear? Is there adequate spacing on the screen or is the screen cluttered and unorganized? Are the graphics clear and of a good size? Is there good contrast in colors? Does the program scroll go too fast or can its speed be controlled by the user? Is sound employed for reinforcement? Are there adequate user support materials and can it be read as is or with a low vision aid?

Large Print Concerns. Are words divided appropriately at the end of a line? Does the program scroll too fast or can its speed be controlled by the user? Is the print large enough for the visually impaired student(s) and clear? Is there adequate spacing on the screen? Is there good contrast in colors? Are the user support materials in large print or is it permissible to enlarge? Are there sound effects utilized for reinforcement? Will the program produce print in various sizes?

Optacon Concerns. Is the print on the screen clear with good contrast? Are there non-standard characters displayed on the screen? Can the user control the speed of the scroll or is it slow enough to be read by the Optacon user? Is there inverse video? (Inverse video can be difficulty to read with the Optacon.) Are the user support materials in braille or on tape? (Reading documentation with the Optacon can be very time-consuming.) Are parts of the program visually dependent — can they be interpreted with an Optacon?

Speech Synthesizer Concerns. Are there pictures, graphics, non-standard characters utilized in the program? (Speech cannot convey the meaning of graphic symbols.) Does the material utilize columns for displaying information? Is there an unusual format that would be difficult to follow if it were presented verbally? Can the speed of speech be controlled? Can it be turned off and on? Does the speech output slow down the student's typing speed? Can the program be used without supervision? Does the program have parts that are visually dependent?

Electronic Braille Concerns. Will the program run with electronic braille devices? Is the information presented in columns? Does the program utilize pictures, graphics, and non-standard characters in the program? Can the scroll speed be controlled by the user? Can the program be modified for use of access devices? Is the reliability of the program changed by the access device? Can the program be used independently by the user? Are parts of the program visually dependent? Can you interrupt and save without having to start completely over each time? Can the program be translated to textfile and then through some braille translation program to braille? (Teacher may want a braille and large print hard copy.) Are there commands that must be entered from the keyboard and cannot be entered for the electronic braille device? Are user support materials available in braille or on tape? Is it permissible to adapt user support materials in braille if they are not available?

SUMMARY

Advances in technology have made many devices for visually impaired and blind persons which help to reduce their handicaps in the area of communication skills. Devices which make information available tactually, auditorially, or in print that is optically, electronically, or physically enlarged was discussed in this chapter. Microcomputers, one of the latest advancements in technology, are becoming valuable educational tools for visually impaired students and were discussed extensively in this chapter.

Visually impaired students use microcomputers for the same purposes as their sighted peers. Because of the varying nature and needs of the visually impaired population, a variety of methods and modes are available to provide access to microcomputers. Most visually impaired students have usable vision and gain access to microcomputers through regular print, enlarged print, and speech synthesis. A smaller percentage of visually impaired students have no usable vision. These students gain access to microcomputers through speech synthesis, electronic braillers, and the Optacon, or a combination of these methods, e.g., a student might regularly use an electronic brailler as an access device, but use an Optacon to read charts.

Two of the major concerns of using microcomputers with visually impaired students are excessive cost and maintenance. Teachers and administrators should be aware of the need to purchase service contracts at the onset so that equipment can be maintained in working condition. Equipment reliability and cost of maintenance should be seriously considered before purchasing any equipment.

Another major concern is the rapidly changing nature of the computer industry (Goodrich, 1984). Students are not quite as affected by the rapidly changing nature of the microcomputer industry as are employees in the business setting. Teachers should assess the needs of each visually impaired student in relation to microcomputers, and purchase equipment to meet their access needs. Students and teachers must realize that just because there is a new and "better" piece of equipment on the market, that doesn't mean that what they are currently using isn't meeting their needs. Too often, we get caught up in the desire to have the latest and best of everything which isn't always feasible or affordable.

CHAPTER 12

INSTRUCTIONAL MATERIALS AND GAMES

THE SELECTION of appropriate materials for use in teaching reading is important in designing individualized educational programs for visually impaired children. Such students may complete the material in a large print or braille basal reading series and may still need more reading and writing opportunities to insure mastery of communication skills. Supplementary books, magazines, reference sources, games, and teaching aids encourage the visually impaired reader to apply reading skills in constructive learning tasks. These materials also offer the reader an opportunity to transfer reading skills to new contexts.

SELECTING INSTRUCTIONAL MATERIALS

A teacher of communications skills, working with students reading braille or enlarged print, is faced with the same constraints as any other teacher in selecting instructional materials. These constraints include cost, storage space, durability, and multi-purpose usage. Due to the large bulk, the excessive cost, and the limited supply of braille and large print materials, these constraints are amplified for the teacher of the visually impaired. In evaluating instructional materials for maximum utility, the following questions might be helpful:

1. Do they meet specific learning needs with measurable results?
2. Are they useful for many students?
3. Are they usable in a variety of contexts?
4. Do they motivate students?
5. Do they require a reasonable amount of teacher instruction and supervision?
6. Do they provide durable service?

Materials Which Meet Specific Learning Needs with Measurable Results

Supplemental reading materials can be effective in teaching children with weaknesses or gaps in specific communication skills. By selecting an activity which focuses on the particular area requiring additional instruction, the teacher can encourage more balanced learning. For example, students having difficulty utilizing initial "th" and "wh" consonant diagraphs to identify words may not need to complete an entire set of phonics lessons focusing on all initial consonant diagraphs, but they can use the time more efficiently with instruction on the deficient skills.

A student having a comprehension problem might utilize materials which focus on simple comprehension skills, such as "locating the answer" or "getting the main idea," through materials designed to emphasize this skill. Materials which present all types of comprehension skills simultaneously might not meet the specific need.

Materials Which Are Useful for Many Students

Teacher preparation or adaptation of materials to meet specific purposes in instruction is essential, yet teachers cannot acquire a different material to teach each skill. Teachers should select materials which will meet needs common to many students. For example, acquiring spelling skills is a problem for braille readers at all age levels. An interesting spelling game or an audible card reader, such as a Language Master or Tutorette, could be used to teach spelling to many braille or large print readers.

Materials Usable in a Variety of Contexts

The experienced teacher may have a favorite store of materials from which to draw for a variety of purposes. For example, cards from a set of Dolch Word Cards, such as those available in braille and large print from the American Printing House, could be used prior to the reading lesson to introduce new vocabulary. The entire set could be used as flash cards to test the student's knowledge of basic sight words and to determine those words which should be included in instruction. Selected words from the set could be used in an activity which requires the student to match words which begin with the same initial consonant or consonant cluster or which contain a common braille contraction. Attempting to acquire separate materials for each of these educational tasks would waste time, money, and storage space.

Materials Which Motivate Students

Perhaps the most valuable attribute of any teaching material is motivation. Although the significance of motivation in braille reading success is well supported in research (Nolan & Kederis, 1969; Olson, Harlow, & Williams, 1975), the motivational value of various instructional materials varies among students. The animal story which intrigues one student may be totally uninteresting to another. Reading materials are needed on a variety of topics. Introducing the visually impaired reader to the many books available through the classroom and library can help the student find materials which can be read with independence and enjoyment.

Materials Which Require a Reasonable Amount of Teacher Instruction and Supervision

Reading instruction through braille or enlarged print is by nature a highly individualized task requiring a great deal of teacher time. Materials may be selected which maximize teacher-student interactions time and eliminate the need for continuous teacher monitoring. Several reading systems, which were programmed for instruction with sighted readers, are available in braille and large print, such as the Barnell Loft Specific Skills Series and Reader's Digest Skills Builders.

The Specific Skills Series deals with eight areas of reading: getting the facts, getting the main idea, locating the answer, detecting a sequence, following directions, drawing conclusions, using the context, and working with sounds. Each area is divided into at least six levels (A-F) and a separate booklet available for each area. Once the teacher determines the student's comprehension needs and reading level, a skills book is selected. After the students get started in the book, they may work almost independently. The materials have the advantage of a consistent format throughout each book so the "students know what to do." The teacher may use the answer key to provide quick teacher feedback or allow the students to check their own work. The American Printing House for the Blind produces more than one such skill series with comparable strands.

Supplementary books, programmed teaching aids, or workbooks should be carefully selected to insure that the student is keeping an appropriate pace and mastering the material rather than only mechanically working through the book. The significance of working independent of teacher supervisoin is equally good for younger readers, because it is the basis of independent study habits.

Materials Which Provide Durable Service

Books and materials used by readers of braille or large print need to be sturdy, because they will receive much handling. Game cards or playing pieces with braille may be made more durable with a thin coat of spray varnish or plastic labeling tape may be used. Large print worksheets or drill cards are more durable if a permanent marking pen rather than a water soluable ink pen is used. Laminated large print materials are more lasting. Instructional materials should be constructed from good raw materials and checked frequently for wear.

Textbooks, supplementary books, periodicals, mechanical teaching aids, and all instructional devices in large print or braille are available from three basic sources: (1) materials designed and produced for the visually impaired, (2) materials produced for normally sighted students but quickly adaptable for use with visually impaired students, and (3) materials made by teachers. A large number of educational materials designed and produced for visually impaired students may be obtained through the American Printing House for the Blind. Other major sources include the American Foundation for the Blind and the Library of the Blind and Physically Handicapped of the Library of Congress. Sources of materials produced for normally sighted students and adapted into braille or large print for visually impaired students are listed in the Central Catalogue of Braille and Large Type Publications that is maintained by the American Printing House for the Blind. A few examples of materials that may be made by the teacher are described below.

GAMES AND ACTIVITIES

The games and independent activities described in this section are specifically designed to help the teacher meet the many individual needs of the visually impaired reader. Many excellent sources of games to reinforce basic reading skills, such as sight word identification, phonics, structural analysis, context clue usage, comprehension of all levels and study skills are available (Spache, 1972b; Olson & Mangold, 1981). Yet, the challenge and complexity of reading with braille or large print may prompt a need for games specifically designed to provide additional instruction. Such activities provide an exciting and motivating setting for reading. Most of the following activities and games can be made easier or more challenging to meet the needs of the student with only a few changes in words or directions. The activities are not labeled by grade level because activities for younger students may be useful for older students with specific needs. Game formats, such as Concentration, Old Maid, Fish Pond, and game boards can be used as the organizational base for reading games. Such activities have the advantage of being familiar to many students and are "time tested" interest stimulators. The following games are illustrative of the types of games that can be used with visually impaired children to assist them in learning reading skills. Some games are designed for the braille reader but most can be adapted for the large print reader.

Pointing Words

The purpose of using this game is to help the reader remember problem words quickly by grouping words in logical clusters. An example is all words beginning with *th*. In braille these are variously represented by *th* = this; *t* = that; dot 5, *the* = there; dots 4, 5, 6, *the* = their; dots 4, 5, *th* = those; dots 4, 5, *the* = these. Each word can be written in braille and large print on braille paper cut in the shape of a pointing hand. The card may be read for quick, accurate recognition and used in games.

1. Simple variations would include making pairs of cards for each word and having students match like words.

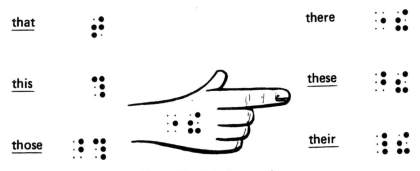

Figure 39. Pointing words.

2. The students draw a point word, read it, and use it correctly in a sentence or provide the full spelling.

3. More challenging games would require students to match pointing words cards with a similar card containing the sentence with the missing words.

Go Fish

The purpose of using this game is to increase reader skills in identifying braille configurations that vary in meaning. Prepare sets of cards which represent each possible use. The meanings of many braille configurations are determined by the position within the line or sentence. For example: dots 2, 5, 6 can be *dis,* "dd," or a period, depending on the location at the first, middle, or end of a word. One card of a set would have written on it the configuration 2, 5, 6, followed immediately by a full cell to represent the initial position. Another would have the same configuration, both preceded and followed by a full cell. The third card would have a full cell followed by the 2, 5, 6 configuration. These three cards would form a matching book of cards. Other books would be made from configurations such as those shown in Figure 40.

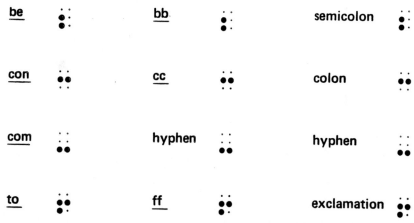

Figure 40. Configurations for Go Fish.

Playing rules for 2 to 4 players follow the familiar rules of Go Fish in which students try to get all cards to make a book by asking for specific cards that the opponent may have. The student with the most books is the prize fisherman. Variations include:

1. Add wild cards with additional meanings which the configuration may have when used as whole word signs.

2. Change to an independent activity for one student, reading through all the cards and matching the books, then supplying a word or sentence in which each is used appropriately.

News Reporter

The use of this game is designed to provide additional practice with the "asking words": why, what, where, who, when, which. Students draw an asking word from a stack of cards. Then each reads a simple story of four or five sentences and looks for the answer to the drawn asking word. At the conclusion of the reading, each reports the question and answer. Variations include:

1. Have the teacher read a challenging story beyond the student's reading level but within comprehension level. Students listen for a particular asking word and indicate by raised hand or tap on the desk when their word is heard.
2. Have students locate asking word in a passage and tally the number of occurrences of each word.

Grade-The-Paper

The objective of this game is to increase skill in proofreading. Prepare several sentences in braille and large print, each containing a designated number of errors which the student must find. The type of errors may be identified at the beginning for all the sentences, such as capitalization and punctuation, or the type of errors to find may change for each sentence or group of sentences. Students read the selection noting the errors. They name each error and identify the correction that should be made. Other variations include:

1. Students state the rule governing the error. A brief summary of rules regrading common errors that students can reference may prompt repeated reading and application of rules.
2. Students may rewrite each sentence correctly. The activity may become a two team game with challenges, penalities, and accumulative scores for each side.

Brain Storm

To foster vocabulary growth and emphasize the relationship between the way a word is spelled and the way it is represented by the braille code, the teacher instructs each pair of players to "brainstorm words" and search for the word containing the most contractions. Examples like "notwithstanding" and "distinguished" might be winners with four contractions each. The pair with the most contractions discovered in one word would win. Variations include:

1. Let students use a dictionary or thesaurus to aid in their search for words.
2. Have students brainstorm for the longest word that is fully spelled in braille. A twelve letter example, such as "redistribute," might be a winner.

Roll-O

This game is designed to help students associate dot numbers with the corresponding braille configurations. Secure or construct six cubes with a different braille numeral on each side (1-6). These cubes are used for playing the game of Roll-O at several levels of difficulty according to the maturity of the players.

For simplest directions, use only two cubes. Players take turns rolling the cubes. The player receives one point for correctly stating any braille character that can be formed by one or both of the numbers (dots). For example, a 2 and a 4 would be the letter "i." If two of the same numbers are rolled such as "2," the student could score by saying "dot 2, comma" and "dot 2, ea." The numeral "5" is the only dot with a single assigned meaning in the literary code. For a roll that results in two "5s," the student might say "dot 5," used in initial letter signs, or be allowed to roll again. Vary the game by rolling more cubes. The player might then score for any possible character correctly begun.

Games designed to emphasize the braille code need not require game boards, puzzles, spinners, or even cards. Many verbal games can be quickly organized and completed and are ideally suited to quickly reward a successful effort or to reinforce a particular skill. In addition, they challenge verbal expression and prompt quick recall. Use letters on each cube instead of numbers, and the large print and braille students may play together. Three cubes, two with consonants and one with vowels, can be used to foster the blending of sounds in short vowel words.

Detecto

The purpose of using this game is to locate and tally the number of times that a designated word, phonic sound, or braille character appears in a sentence or passage. The teacher asks the student to go on a detective hunt. The student may scan a short selection and visually or tactually locate a new vocabulary word prior to reading the passage. In this fashion the student is having multiple opportunities to see the new word. The various forms of the word (e.g., with a capital letter next to punctuation) may be discussed in advance. Several students may be involved.

With a braille contraction such as the "ed" sign, the student may read a sentence such as: "Ned played with his red wagon." and find the character three times: N*ed*, play*ed*, and r*ed*. The teacher may assign each student a different word or braille character.

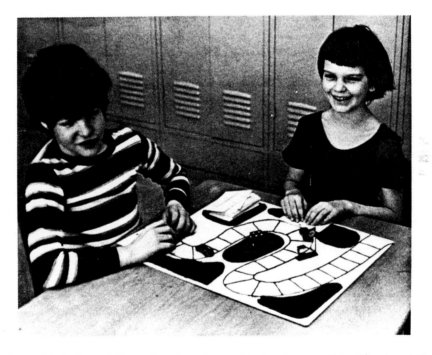

Figure 41. A Tactual Game Board can be used to develop word identification skills.

Tactual Game Board

This game is designed to develop sight word identification skills. The tactual game board can be used to foster a variety of other reading activities (see Figure 41). Some boards that are commercially available may be made tactual through the addition of string, felt, and yarn. Others are not suitable for adaptation because of clutter or intricate patterns. A durable magnetic game board may be made from a metal cookie sheet or stove protector. String or yarn may be glued to make a ladder-like track with twenty to thirty spaces. A graphic package with a computer and braille printer may make other tactual games. Small magnetic objects can be used as markers for each player. Players draw cards in turn and read the sentences or words. The student may check an answer with the teacher or if two students are playing independently, they may assume cards are read correctly if both concur that the word is correct. Players read cards alternately and each moves in turn. A missed word means a lost turn.

Many variations increase the use of a game board:

1. Each player may have separate stacks of word or phrase cards to allow for individual differences.
2. Once the teacher has introduced and supervised the game, it may become an independent activity for special rewards. Lengthen the suspense for experienced players of the game by inserting cards which say "skip two spaces" or "go back one block."
3. To determine the number of moves each player may take, let each have a turn to spin, using a spinner with braille and large print numerals, indicating the length of the move.
4. A wooden cube with numerals on each side becomes a dice to roll to determine the length of the move. Number names may be substituted for numerals.
5. Several sets of cards allow the game to serve many instructional purposes. Ideally, cards from the student's vocabulary, homonyms, compound words, synonyms, or words to be analyzed phonetically, which are used for other purposes, can be used in the board game.

Sorting Trays

This game will help to provide visually impaired students with a method to organize and manipulate cards and objects for independent activities. Sectional trays can provide organization for a variety of reading activities. Presectioned trays are commercially available or sections can be made in trays by the addition of wood or plastic strips cut and glued in place.

A reading readiness activity might introduce pairing material pieces of the same texture. Other variations include:

1. Students may match small objects with a card showing the initial letter or name.

2. The tray may be used to group many small objects of the same initial sound.

3. It may also be used to group similar contractions at an upper elementary level. The student may be presented with some words in the tray and asked to sort additional words containing the same contractions, regardless of where the contraction falls in the word.

The Long and Short

The purpose of using this game is to provide practice in finding vowel sounds and in comparing the sound to the symbol. Students make up sentences of five words, using each vowel sound once in the sentence. The students tell their sentence and designate whether each vowel is long or short and where the vowel appears. An example might be:

"Red gave it to us."

e   a   i o u

In the braille sentence the letters "e," "i," and "o" do not actually appear in the written braille format since they are represented by the contraction in braille. Vary the game by requiring all long or all short vowels such as in the example:

"You go away each night."

u o a   e   i

Fish Pond

The objective of using this game is to teach new sight words and to review old ones. The teacher may prepare or purchase fish-shaped word cards with high frequency words. Each fish-card could have a washer glued on for an "eye." A stick and string with a magnet tied to the end of the string make a fishing pole. The student fishes for a fish card and then reads the word on the fish. The student keeps the fish read correctly and must throw back those missed. Other suggestions include:

1. Let students construct as many phrases as possible from the fish cards.

2. Include in the pond only words of a particular contraction or phonetic type, such as alphabet word signs or long vowel words.

3. Ask students to identify the word in braille and then provide the full spelling.

Cloze Stories

This game is designed to increase the student's use of context clues to identify words. Some words in the story may be covered or omitted. The teacher may construct a short passage in which all single cell words are covered by a flap of paper taped over the word. Ask students to read the passage and predict appropriate words. Then let them check their predictions by lifting each flap and reading the original word. Score one point for a prediction that makes language sense. Score two points for a prediction which exactly matches the text. All such passages should contain only words which the student can read easily. To be able to predict from the context the student must identify the surrounding words. A sample passage might read:

_____ turtle _____ walking slowly around _____ old log. Suddenly _____ head _____ feet slipped into _____ shell.

1. Change the game by deleting different contracted forms such as multiple cell contractions or lower signs.

2. Omit only nouns or verbs and retain the first letter in each to aid in identification:

The b____ heard his d____ barking as a big fire t____ raced down the r____ .

Riddles

This game will help to review braille contractions and rules for usage. The teacher may prepare riddles that require the player to identify the contraction in the riddle and also tell why it appears in some of the words but not in others. The following riddle is an example:

You'll find me in "cream" also in "treating;"
In "bread," but never in "eating."
Answer: "ea" used in the the middle of a word, but not in "eating" because "ea" cannot be used at beginning of a word.

We may be known as the favorite five:
With pride we are ready to burst,
For if we're even involved in a choice,
We'll be certain to come out first.
Answer: "and," "for," "with," "of," "the" take preference over all other contractions if they save as much space as the alternative.

Let someone else start and we'll follow along,
But we never like to lead the way;

Just once in awhile we move off alone
When there is not enough room to stay.

Answer: (two choices) final letter signs: "ble" and "ing." None of the final letter signs can be used to start a word.

Object File

This activity is designed to teach letter sounds. The teacher may develop an object file, or collection of many small objects. To construct an object file, many objects are collected from home and school and grouped in boxes according to the initial consonant sounds. The objects or models may be used as a picture file for blind or sighted students. Once the file is begun, it can be adapted for story illustrations, games, rhyming words, manipulative, classifying, and matching activities. It can serve as a storage system for common classroom objects such as scissors, tape, and crayons, encouraging utilization of initial consonant sounds in locating objects and returning them to the correct box. Students can help fill the boxes by adding paper to the "p" box, cups to the "c" box, etc.

A file of many small models and objects, Tactual Aids to Reading, is available commercially through the American Printing House for the Blind. Included are objects representing all initial alphabet sounds and a teacher's manual of suggested activities. Through the object file the teacher can insure that the visually impaired student has had tactual experience with common small objects, such as pliers, screwdriver, can opener, feathers, cork, etc. Variations include:

1. At a readiness level, have students sort objects into the appropriate box by the initial consonant sound beginning with sharply contrasting consonant sounds, such as /p/ and /n/ or /t/ and /k/.
2. For beginning readers prepared word cards for the objects and let students pair objects and words.
3. Have students sort objects by function, such as tools (pliers, wrench, screwdriver, hammer) or tableware (plate, cup, fork, knife, spoon).
4. Separate boxes may be made for initial digraphs (sh, th, wh, ch) and consonant clusters (s-blends, l-blends, r-blends).

SUMMARY

Teachers presented with the challenge of providing reading instruction through braille or large print will need materials and activities beyond those contained in the basic reader series. Supplemental reading materials may be found in the form of library books, periodicals, reference sources, and games. Reading materials should be carefully selected to meet specific learning needs as well as to be versatile, compact, sturdy, and motivating. The several games presented in this chapter are a sampling of the many activities which can supplement reading instruction.

REFERENCES

American Association of Instructors of the Blind. (1853). *Proceedings of the First Convention*. Batavia, NY: Office of Spirit of Times.

American Association of Instructors of the Blind. (1871). *Proceedings of the Second Convention*. Indianapolis, IN: Indianapolis Printing and Publishing House.

American Printing House for the Blind. (1986). *Distribution of Federal Quota Based on the January 7, 1985 Registration of Eligible Students*. Louisville, KY: American Printing House for the Blind.

Anderson, D. W. (1984). Mental imagery in congenitally blind children. *Journal of Visual Impairment and Blindness, 78*(5), 206-210.

Anderson, D. W., & Fischer, K. P. (1986). Nominal realism in congenitally blind children. *Journal of Visual Impairment and Blindness, 80*(8), 896-900.

Anderson, D. W., & Olson, M. R. (1981). Word meaning among congenitally blind children. *Journal of Visual Impairment and Blindness, 75*(4), 165-168.

Anderson, T. (May, 1980). Microfiche as a reading aid for partially sighted students. *Journal of Visual Impairment and Blindness, 74*(5), 193-196.

Ashcroft, S. C. (1960). *Errors in oral reading of braille at elementary grade levels*. Unpublished doctoral dissertation. Urbana, IL: University of Illinois.

Ashcroft, S. C. (Winter, 1984). Research on multimedia access to microcomputers for visually impaired youth. *Education of the Visually Handicapped, 15*(4), 108-118.

Ashcroft, S. C., Halliday, S., & Barraga, N. (1965). *Effects of experimental teaching on the visual behavior of children educated as though they had no vision*. U. S. Office of Education Grant No. 32-52-120-1034. Nashville: George Peabody College for Teachers.

Ashcroft, S. C., & Young M. (1981). Microcomputers for visually impaired and multihandicapped persons. *Journal of Special Education Technology, 4*(2), 24-27.

Aulls, M. W. (1982). Developing reading in today's elementary school. Boston: Allyn & Bacon.

Baratz, J. C., & Shuy, R. W. (Eds.). (1969). *Teaching black children to read*. Washington, DC: Center for Applied Linguistics.

Barraga, N. C. (1964). *Increased visual behavior in low vision children*. Research Series No. 13. New York: American Foundation for the Blind.

Barraga, N. C. (1970). *Visual Efficiency Scale*. Louisville: American Printing House for the Blind.

Barraga, N. C. (1976). Visual handicaps and learning: A developmental approach. Belmont, CA: Wadsworth.

Barraga, N. C., Dorward, B., & Ford, P. (1973). *Aids for teaching basic concepts of sensory development.* Louisville: American Printing House for the Blind.

Barraga, N. C., & Morris, J. E. (1980). *Programs to develop efficiency in visual functioning.* Louisville: American Printing House for the Blind.

Best, H. (1919). *The blind.* New York: The MacMillan Company.

Betts, E. A. (1967). *Foundations of reading instructions (with emphasis on differentiated guidance).* New York: American Book Company.

Birch, J. W., Tisdall, W. J., Peabody, R. L., & Sterrett, R. (1966). *School achievement and effect of type size on reading in visually handicapped children.* Program in Special Education and Rehabilitation, Cooperative Research Project #1766, School of Education. Pittsburg: University of Pittsburg.

Bischoff, R. W. (1967). Improvement of listening comprehension in partially sighted students. *Sight-Saving Review, 37*(3), 161-164.

Bischoff, R. W. (1979). Listening: A teachable skills for visually impaired persons. *Journal of Visual Impairment and Blindness, 73*(2), 59-68.

Bloomfield, L., & Barnhart, C. L. (1961). *Let's read — A linguistic approach.* Detroit: Wayne State University Press.

Boehm, A. E. (1971). Boehm test of basic concepts (test manual). New York: The Psychological Corporation.

Bond, G. L., & Dykstra, R. (1967). The cooperative research program in first-grade reading instruction. *Reading Research Quarterly, 2*(4), 5-142.

Bortner, M. (1985). Review of Wechsler Intelligence Scale for Children. In J. V. Mitchell (Ed.), *The Ninth Mental Measurements Yearbook.* Lincoln, NB: Univeristy of Nebraska.

Bradfield, A. L. (1984). Low vision aids. In R. K. Harley & G. A. Lawrence (Eds.), *Visual impairment in the schools.* Springfield, IL: Charles C Thomas.

Brand, H. J. (1976). The use of closed-circuit television as an aid in the administration of psychological tests to partially sighted children. *Education of the Visually Handicapped, 8*(2), 53-57.

Bruce, R. E. (May, 1973). Using the overhead projector with visually impaired students. *Education of the Visually Handicapped, 5*(2), 43-46.

Bruner, J. (1975). The ontogenesis of speech acts. *Journal of Child Language, 2*(1), 1-9.

Brunken, P. (1984). Independence for the visually handicapped through technology. *Education of the Visually Handicapped, 15*(4), 127-135.

Budoff, M., & Hutten, L. R. (1982). Microcomputers in special education: Promises and pitfalls, *Exceptional Children, 49*(2), 123-128.

Buell, C. E. (1966). *Physical education for blind children.* Springfield, IL: Charles C Thomas.

Burklen, K. (1932). *Touch reading of the blind.* New York: American Foundation for the Blind.

Burns, P. C. (1980). *Assessment and correction of language arts difficulties.* Columbus: Charles E. Merrill.

Carter, B. (1962). How to use educational recordings effectively: A survey of blind college students. *New Outlook for the Blind, 56*(9), 332-334.

Caton, H. R. (1974). Tactual aids for reading: Guidelines for Teachers. Louisville: American Printing House for the Blind.

Caton, H. R. (1977). The development of a tactile analog to the Boehm test of basic concepts, form A. *Journal of Visual Impairments and Blindness, 71*(9), 382-386.

Chaffin, G., Maxwell, B., & Thompson, B. (1982). *Academic skill builders.* Allen, TX: Development Learning Materials.

Chall, J. S. (1967). *Learning to read: The great debate.* New York: McGraw.

Cholden, L. S. (1958). *A psychiatrist works with blindness.* New York: American Foundation for the Blind.

Cobb, E. S. (1977). Learning through listening: A new approach. *Journal of Visual Impairment and Blindness, 71*(5), 302-308.

Cohoe, E. (1961). Typewriting for partially seeing and blind children. *Exceptional Children, 28,* 13-17.

Craig, R. H. (1975). A personal approach to teaching braille to youths and adults. *New Outlook for the Blind,* 69, 11-19.

Crandell, J. M., & Wallace, D. H. (1974). Speed reading in braille: An empirical study. *New Outlook for the Blind, 68*(1), 13-19.

Cratty, B. J. (1971). *Movement and spatial awareness in blind children and youth.* Springfield, IL: Charles C Thomas.

Cratty, B. J., & Sams, R. S. (1968). *The body image of blind children.* New York: American Foundation for the Blind.

Crosby, R. M., & Liston, R. A. (1976). *The waysiders: Reading and the dyslexic child.* New York: John Day Company.

Cutsforth, T. D. (1951). The blind in school and society: A psychological study. New York: American Foundation for the Blind.

Dale, P. S. (1972). *Language development: Structure and function.* Hinsdale, IL: Dryden Press.

Davidson, P. W., Wiles-Kettenmann, M., Haber, R. N., & Appelle, S. (1980). Relationship between hand movements, reading competence, and passage difficulty in braille reading. *Neuropschologia, 18,* 629-635.

Deno, S. L. (1985). Curriculum-based measurement: The emerging alternative. *Exceptional Child, 52*(3), 219-232.

Deshler, D. O. (1978). Psychoeducational aspects of learning disabled adolescents. In L. Mann, L. Goodman, & J. L. Wiederholt (Eds.), *Teaching the learning disabled adolescent.* Boston: Houghton-Mifflin.

Dibble, F. J. B. (1984). Focus on the hands: A beginning approach to teaching typing to visually impaired, multiply handicapped students. *Journal of Visual Impairment and Blindness, 78*(8), 345-349.

Dolch, E. W., (1950). *Teaching primary reading.* Champaign: Garrard.

Dorward, B., & Barraga, N. (1968). *Teaching aids for blind and visually limited children.* New York: American Foundation for the Blind.

Duckworth, E. (1979). Either we're too early and they can't learn it or we're too late and they know it already: The dilemma of "applying Piaget?" *Harvard Educational Review, 49,* 297-312.

Duncan, B. (1969). *Touch and tell.* Louisville: American Printing House for the Blind.

Dupress, J. K. (1963). Summary of preceedings of the International Congress on Technology and Blindness. In L. Clark (Ed.), *Proceedings of the International Congress on Technology and Blindness.* New York: American Foundation for the Blind.

Durr, W. K. (1973). Computer study of high frequency words in popular trade juveniles. *The Reading Teacher, 27,* 37-42.

Eakin, W. M., & McFarland, T. L. (1960). *Type, printing and the partially seeing child.* Pittsburgh: Stanwix.

Eatman, P. F. (1942). An analytic study of braille reading. Unpublished doctoral dissertation, University of Texas.

Epstein, H. (1986). Multimodality, crosmodality, and dyslexia. *Annals of Dyslexia, 35.*

Ethington, D. (1956). The readability of braille as a function of three spacing variables. Master's Thesis, University of Kentucky.

Evans, R., & Simpkins, K. (1972). Computer assisted instruction for the blind. *Education of the Visually Handicapped, 4*(3), 83-85.

Farnham-Diggory, S. (1978). *Learning disabilities: A psychological perspective.* Cambridge, MA: Harvard University Press.

Farrell, G. (1956). *The story of blindness.* Cambridge: Harvard University Press.

Fernald, G. M. (1943). *Remedial techniques for basic school subjects.* New York: McGraw Hill.

Ferrell, K. A. (1985). *Reach out and teach.* New York: American Foundation for the Blind.

Fertsch, P. (1946). An analysis of braille reading. *Outlook for the Blind and Teachers Forum, 40,* 128-131.

Flanigan, P. J., & Joslin, E. S. (1969). Patterns of response in the perception of braille configuration. *New Outlook for the Blind, 63*(8), 232-244.

Foreman, D. (1983). Search of the literature. In D. O. Harper & J. H. Stewarts (Eds.), *RUN: Computer Education.* Monterey, CA; Brooks/Cole Publishing Company.

Fortell, E. R. (1985). The case for conservative reader placement. *Reading Teacher, 38*(9), 857-862.

Foulke, E. (1966). Comparison of comprehension of two forms of compressed speech. *Exceptional Children, 33,* 169-173.

Foulke, E. (1979). Investigative approaches to the study of braille reading. *Journal of Visual Impairment and Blindness, 73,* 298-308.

Foulke, E. (1981). Impact of science and technology on the early years. *Journal of Visual Impairment and Blindness, 75*(3), 101-108.

Fraiberg, S. (1977). Insights from the blind: Comparative studies of blind and sighted infants. New York: Basic Books Inc.

Fraiberg, S., Siegel, B. L., & Gibson, R. (1966). The role of sound in the search behavior of the blind infant. In R. S. Eissler et al. (Eds.), *The psychoanalytic study of the child, 21,* 327-357. New York: International Universities Press.

Frampton, M. E., & Kerney, E. (1953). *The residential school.* New York: New York Institute for the Education of the Blind.

Frampton, M. E., & Rowell, H. G. (1938). *Education of the handicapped.* Vol. I. Yonkers-on-Hudson, NY: World Book Company.

Frederikesen, J., Warren, B., Gillote, H., & Weaver, P. (1982). The name of the game is literacy. *Classroom Computer News,* May/June, 23-27.

French, R. S. (1932). *From Homer to Helen Keller.* New York: American Foundation for the Blind.

Freund, E. (1968). Screen pads for long-hand writing. *New Outlook for the Blind, 62,* 144-147.

Freund, E. D. (1970). Long-hand writing for the blind. Louisville, KY: American Printing House for the Blind.

Fries, C. C. (1963). *Linguistics and Reading.* New York: HR&W.

Fry, E. B. (1972). *Reading instruction for the classroom and clinic.* New York: McGraw.

Furness, E. L. (1955). A remedial and developmental program in listening. *Elementary English, 32,* 525-531.

Garry, R. J., & Ascarelli, A. (1960). Teaching topographical orientation and spatial orientation to congenitally blind children. *Journal of Education, 143*(2), 1-48.

Gates, A. I. (1922). Psychology of reading and spellng with special reference to disability. *Contributions to Education,* 129, Teachers College, Columbia University.

Gates, A. I. (1931). *Interest and ability in reading.* New York: MacMillan.

Genshaft, J. L., Dare, N. L., & O'Malley, P. L. (1980). Assessing the visually impaired child: A school psychology view. *Journal of Visual Impairment and Blindness, 74,* 344-350.

Gibson, E. J. (1969). *Principles of perceptual learning and development.* Englewood Cliffs, NJ: Prentice Hall.

Gill, J. M. (1983). *International survey of aids for the visually disabled* (3rd edition). Oxbridge, England: Brunel University.

Gillingham, A., & Stillman, B. W. (1960). *Remedial techniques for children and specific disability in reading, spelling, and penmanship* (6th edition). New York: Lithographing Corporation.

Gleason, D. (1984). Auditory assessment of visually impaired preschoolers: A team effort. *Education of the Visually Handicapped, 16*(3), 102-113.

Goldish, L. H., & Taylor, H. E. (1974). The Optacon: A valuable device for blind persons. *The New Outlook for the Blind, 63*(2), 49-56.

Goldman, R., Fristoe, M., & Woodcock, R. W. (1974). Goldman-Fristoe-Woodcock diagnostic auditory discrimination test. Circle Pines, MN: American Guidance Service.

Goodman, K. S., (Ed.). (1973). *Miscue analysis is applications to reading instruction.* Urbana: ERIC/RCS, National Council of Teachers of English.

Goodrich, G. L. (1984). Application of microcomputers by visually impaired persons. *Journal of Visual Impairment and Blindness, 78*(9), 408-414.

Goodrich, G. L., Bennett, R., De L'aune, W. R., Lauer, H., & Mowinski, L. (1979). Kurzweil reading machine: a partial evaluation of its optical character recognition error rate. *Journal of Visual Impairment and Blindness, 73*(10), 389-399.

Grimes, L. (1981). Computers are for kids: Designing software programs to avoid problems of learning. *Teaching Exceptional Children, 14* (2), 48-53.

Hall, A., & Rodabaugh, B. (1979). Development of a pre-reading concept program for visually handicapped children. *Journal of Visual Impairment and Blindness, 73*(7), 257-263.

Hallahan, D. P., & Kauffman, J. M. (1976). *Introduction to learning disabilities: A psychobehavioral approach.* Englewood Cliffs, NJ: Prentice-Hall.

Halliday, C. (1970). *The visually impaired child: Growth learning, development — Infancy to school age.* Louisville, KY: American Printing House for the Blind.

Hamilton, C. A. (1910). Association of Instructors of the Blind. *Twenty-first Biennial Convention*. Little Rock: Arkansas School for the Blind.

Hanna, P. R., Hodges, R. E., & Hanna, J. S. (1971). *Spelling: Structure and strategies*. Boston: Houghton Mifflin.

Hannaford, A. E. (1983). Microcomputers in special education: Some new opportunities, some old problems. *The Computing Teacher, 10*(6), 11-17.

Hannaford, A. E., & Sloan, E. (1981). Microcomputers: Powerful learning tools with proper programming. *Teaching Exceptional Children, 14*(2), 54-57.

Hargis, C. H. (1982). Word recognition development. *Focus on Exceptional Children, 14*(9), 1-8.

Hargrove, L. J., & Poteet, J. G. (1984). *Assessment in special education*. Englewood Cliffs: Prentice-Hall.

Haring, N. G., & Phillips, E. L. (1972). *Analysis and modification of classroom behavior*. Englewood Cliffs, MJ: Prentice-Hall.

Harley, R. K. (1963). Verbalism among blind children: *An investigation and analysis*. Research Series No. 10. New York: American Foundation for the Blind.

Harley, R. K., & Lawrence, G. A. (1984). *Visual impairment in the schools*. Springfield, IL: Charles C Thomas.

Harley, R. K., Pichert, J. W., & Morrison, M. (1985). Braille instruction for blind diabetic adults with decreased tactile sensitivity. *Journal of Visual Impairment and Blindness, 79*(1), 12-17.

Harley, R. K., Pichert, J. W., & Morrison, M. B. (1986). Teaching braille reading to tactially impaired blind adults with diabetes: Case report. *The Diabetes Education, 12*, 43-47.

Harley, R. K., & Rawls, R. (1970). Comparison of several approaches for teaching braille reading to blind chldren. *Education of the Visually Handicapped, 2*, 47-51.

Harley, R. K., & Long, R., (1986). *The development of a program in orientation and mobility for multiply impaired blind infants*. Field Initiated Research Project, Final Report to U. S. Department of Education.

Harley, R. K., Wood, T. A., & Merbler, J. B. (1975). Programmed instruction in orientation and mobility for multiply impaired children. *The New Outlook for the Blind, 69*(9), 418-423.

Hathaway, W. (1959). *Education and health of the partially seeing child* (4th edition). New York: National Society for the Prevention of Blindness.

Hayes, S. P. (1918). Report of a preliminary test of the reading of the pupils of the Pennsylvania Institution for the Instruction of the Blind at Overbrook, Pennsylvania. *The Outlook for the Blind, 12*, 1-20.

Hayes, S. D. (1920). The work of the Department of Psychological Research at the Pennsylvania Institution for the Instruction of the Blind, Overbrook. *The Outlook for the Blind, 14*, 5-20.

Heasley, B. E. (1974). *Auditory perceptual disorders and remediation*. Springfield, IL: Charles C Thomas.

Hegge, T. G., Kirk, S. A., & Kirk, W. (1973). *Remedial reading drills*. Ann Arbor, MI: George Wahr Publishing Company.

Henderson, F. M. (1967). The effects of character recognition training on braille reading. Unpublished specialist in education thesis, Nashville, George Peabody College for Teachers.

Henderson, F. M. (1973). Communication skills. In B. Lowenfeld (Ed.), *The visually handicapped child in school.* New York: The John Day Company.

Hendrickson, W. B. (1972). *From shelter to self-reliance: A history of the Illinois Braille and Sight Saving School.* Jacksonville: Illinois Braille and Sight Saving School.

Henrichs, R., & Moorhouse, J. (1969). Touch perception thresholds in blind diabetic subjects in relation to the reading of braille type. *New England Journal of Medicine, 280,* 72-76.

Hill, E. W. (1981). The Hill Performance Test of selected positional concepts. Chicago: Stoelting Company.

Hill, E. W. (1986). Orientation and mobility. In G. T. Scholl (Ed.), *Foundations of Education for Blind and Visually Handicapped Children and Youth,* 315-340. New York: American Foundation for the Blind.

Hofmeister, A. M. (1982). Microcomputers in perspective. *Exceptional Children, 49*(2), 115-121.

Holland, B. G. (1934). Speed and pressure factors in braille reading. *Teachers Forum, 7,* 13-17.

Huckins, A. (1965). Teaching handwriting to the blind student. *The New Outlook for the Blind, 59*(2), 63-65.

Illingworth, W. H. (1910). *History of the education of the blind.* London: Sampson Low, Marston and Company.

Illinois Braille Committee. (1983). *Braille Series 1060.* Louisville: American Printing House for the Blind.

Irwin, R. B. (1955). *As I Saw It.* New York: American Foundation for the Blind.

Israel, L. (1973). CCTV reading machines for visually handicapped persons: A guide for selection. *The New Outlook for the Blind, 67*(3), 102-110.

Jankowski, L. W., & Evans, J. K. (1981). The exercise capacity of blind children. *Journal of Visual Impairment and Blindness, 75,* 248-251.

Johnson, D. D. (1971). The Dolch list re-examined. *The Reading Teacher, 24,* 455-456.

Johnson, D. J., & Myklebust, H. R. (1967). *Learning disabilities: Educational principles and practices.* New York: Grune & Stratton.

Joiner, L. M., Sedlak, R. A., Silverstein, B. J., & Densel, G. (1980). Microcomputers: An available technology for special education. *Journal of Special Education Technology, 3*(2), 37-42.

Jose, R. J. (1983). *Understanding low vision.* New York: American Foundation for the Blind.

Kershman, S. M. (1976). A hierarchy of tasks in the development of tactual discrimination (Part 1). *Education of the Visually Handicapped, 8*(3), 73-82.

Kirk, S. A., McCarthy, J. J., & Kirk, W. D. (1968). *Illinois test of psycholinguistic abilities* (Rev. ed.). Urbana: University of Illinois Press.

Kirk, S. A., Kliebhan, J. M., & Lerner, J. W. (1978). Teaching reading to slow and disabled learners. Boston: Houghton Mifflin.

Koenig, A. J., Mack, C. G., Schenk, W. A. & Ashcroft, S. C. (1985). Developing writing and word processing skills with visually impaired children: A beginning. *Journal of Visual Impairment and Blindness, 79*(7), 308-312.

Krebs, B. M. (1968). *Braille in brief.* Louisville: American Printing House for the Blind.

Krebs, B. M. (1973). *ABC's of braille.* Louisville: American Printing House for the Blind.

Kurzhals, I. W. (1966). Reading made meaningful through a readiness for learning program. *International Journal for the Education of the Blind, 15*(4), 107-111.

Kurzhals, I. W., & Caton, H. (1974). *A tactual road to reading: Developmental program for young children.* Louisville: American Printing House for the Blind.

Kusajima, T. (1974). *Visual reading and braille reading: An experimental investigation of the physiology and psychology of visual and tactual reading.* (Clark, L. L., & Jastrembska, Z. S., Ed.) New York: American Foundation for the Blind.

Langley, M. B. (1980). *Functional vision inventory.* Chicago: Stoelting.

Langley, M. B. (1986). Psychoeducational assessment of visually impaired students with additional handicaps. In D. Ellis (Ed.), *Sensory impairments in mentally handicapped people.* Beckenham, KY: Croom Helm Ltd.

LaSasso, C. M., & Jones, T. W. (1984). A survey of approaches to teaching reading to visually impaired students in residential schools. *Journal of Visual Impairments and Blindness, 78*(6), 263-264.

Lowenfeld, B. (1975). *The changing status of the blind.* Springfield: Charles C Thomas.

Lowenfeld, B. (1973). *The visually handicapped child in school.* New York: John Day.

Lowenfeld, B., Abel, G. L., & Hatlen, P. H. (1969). *Blind children learn to read.* Springfield: Charles C Thomas.

Lundstein, S. W. (1979). *Listening, its impact at all levels on reading and the other language arts.* Urbana, IL: ERIC Clearinghouse on Reading and Communication Skills, National Institute of Education.

Mack, C. (1984). How useful is braille? Reports of Blind Adults. *Journal of Visual Impairment and Blindness, 78*(7), 311-313.

Malone, T. W. (1981). What makes computer games fun? *BYTE,* 258-277.

Mangieri, J. N., & Kahn, M. S. (1977). Is the Dolch list of basic sight words irrelevant? *The Reading Teacher, 30*(6), 649-651.

Mangold, S. (1978). Tactile perception and braille letter recognition: Effects of developmental teaching. *Journal of Visual Impairment and Blindness, 72*(7), 259-266.

Marks, A., & Marks, R. (1956). *Teaching the blind script-writing by the marks method.* New York: American Foundation for the Blind.

Maxfield, K. E. (1928), *The blind child and his reading.* New York: American Foundation for the Blind.

Mellor, M. (1979). Technical innovations in braille reading, writing, and production. *Journal of Visual Impairment and Blindness, 73*(8), 339-341.

Mercer, C. D., & Mercer A. (1985). *Teaching students with learning problems* (2nd ed.). Columbus, OH: Charles Merrill.

Millar, S. (1975). Spatial memory by blind and sighted children. *British Journal of Psychology, 66*(4), 449-459.

Millar, S. (1978). Short-term serial tactual recall: Effects of grouping on tactually probed recall of braille letters and nonsense shapes by blind children. *British Journal of Psychology, 69*(1), 17-24.

Miller, D. D. (1985). Reading comes naturally: A mother and her blind child's experiences. *Journal of Visual Impairment and Blindness, 79*(1), 1-4.

Miller, G. A. (1983). Computers in education: A non-Orwellian view. In D. O. Harper & J. H. Stewarts (Eds.), *RUN: Computer Education.* Monterey, CA: Brookes/Cole Publishing Company.

Mills, A. E. (1983). The acquisition of speech sounds in the visually handicapped child. In A. E. Mills (Ed.), *Language acquisition in the blind child: Normal and deficient.* San Diego: College Hill Press.

Mills, R. J. (1970). Orientation and mobility for teachers. *Education of the Visually Handicapped, 2*(3), 80-82.

Mommers, M. J. C. (1976). Braille reading: Factors affecting achievement of Dutch elementary school childen. *New Outlook for the Blind, 70*(8), 332-340.

Monroe, M. (1951). *Growing into reading.* Chicago: Scott F.

Morgan, J. H. (1975). *Computer-assisted instruction for the blind and deaf.* Cincinnati: Cincinnati Public Schools, ERIC Document Reproduction Service No. ED 107 039.

Morris, J. E. (1966). Relative efficiency of reading and listening for braille and large type readers. In 48th American Biennial Conference of the American Association of Instructors of bhe Blind. Washington, DC: American Association of Instructors for the Blind.

Morris, J. E. (1974). The 1973 Stanford Achievement Test series as adopted for use by the visually handicapped. *Education of the Visually Handicapped, 6*(2), 33-43.

Morris, J. E. (1976). Facilitating the education of the visually handicapped through research in communications, Part One. Facilitating Listening as a Medium for Education of the Visually Impaired Grant No. OEG-0-73-0642, U. S. Office of Education. Louisville: American Printing House for the Blind.

Morris, J. E. (1976). Adaptation of the Durrell listening-reading series for use with visually handicapped. *Education of the Visually Handicapped, 8*(1), 21-27.

Morris, J. E., & Hill, D. G. (1976). A consumer review of cassette dictionary. In final report, Grant No. OEG-0-73-0642, U. S. Office of Education. Facilitating the Education of the Visually Handicapped through Research in Communications, June Morris, Editor. Louisville: American Printing House for the Blind.

National Library Service for the Blind and Physically Handicapped. (1986). *Library resources for the blind and physically handicapped.* Washington, DC: Library of Congress.

Newman, S. E., & Hall, A. D. (1986). Amount learned from two alphabets used with the blind. In annual meeting of the Eastern Psychological Association, New York, NY.

Nolan, C. Y. (1959). Readability of large type: A study of type sizes and type styles. *International Journal for the Education of the Blind, 9*(2), 41-44.

Nolan, C. Y. (1963). Reading and listening in learning by the blind. *Exceptional Children, 29*(7), 313-316.

Nolan, C. Y. (1966). *Reading and listening in learning by the blind.* Unpublished report. Louisville: American Printing House for the Blind.

Nolan, C. Y., & Kederis, C. J. (1969). *Perceptual factors in braille word recognition* (AFB Research Series No. 20). New York: American Foundation for the Blind.

Nolan, C. Y., & Morris, J. E. (1969). Learning by blind students through active and passive listening. *Exceptional Children, 36*(3), 173-181.

Nolan, C. Y., & Morris, J. E. (1973). Final report, Grant No. OEG-0-8-080046-2670(032). *Aural Study Systems for the Visually Handicapped,* U. S. Office of Education. Louisville: American Printing House for the Blind.

Northern, J. L., & Downs, M. T. (1974). *Hearing in children.* Baltimore: Williams and Wilkins.

Oakland, T., & Williams, F. C. (1971). *Auditory perception.* Seattle: Special Child Publications.

Okey, J. R. (1976). Diagnostic testing pays off. *Science Teacher, 43,* 27.

Olson, M. R. (1977). Teaching faster braille reading in the primary grades. *Journal of Visual Impairment and Blindness, 7*(3), 122-124.

Olson, M. R., Harlow, S. D., & Williams, J. (1975). Rapid reading in braille and large print: An examination of McBride's procedures. *New Outlook for the Blind, 69*(9), 392-395.

Olson, M. R., & Mangold, S. (1981). *Guidelines and games for teaching efficient braille reading.* New York: American Foundation for the Blind.

Oreton, S. R. (1937). *Reading, writing, and speech problems in children.* New York: Norton.

Pearson, M. A. (1963). The establishment of school and college ability test norms for blind children in grades 4, 5, and 6. *International Journal of Education of the Blind, 12*(4), 110-112.

Piaget, J. (1969). *Science of education and psychology of the child.* New York: Viking Press.

Polloway, E. A., Patton, J. R., & Cohen, S. B. (1981). Written language for mildly handicapped students. *Focus on Exceptional Children, 14*(3).

Pring, L. (1985). Processes involved in braille reading. *Journal of Visual Impairment and Blindness, 79*(6), 252-255.

Revesz, G. (1950). *Psychology and art of the blind.* Translated by H. A. Wolff. New York: Longman.

Restak, R. (1984). *The brain.* New York: Bantam Books.

Ross, A. O. (1977). *Learning disability: The unrealized potential.* New York: McGraw-Hill.

Rossi, P. (1980). Closed circuit television — a method of reading. *Education of the Visually Handicapped, 12*(3), 90-94.

Ruconich, S. (1984). Evaluating microcomputer access technology for use by visually impaired students. *Education of the Visually Handicapped, 15*(4), 119-125.

Ryan, S. G., & Bedi, D. N. (1978). Toward computer literacy for visually impaired students. *Journal of Visual Impairment and Blindness, 72*(8), 302-306.

Salvia, J., & Ysseldyke, J. E. (1981). *Assessment in special and remedial education.* Boston: Houghton Mifflin Company.

Sanford, L. (1984). A formative evaluation of an instructional program designed to teach visually impaired students to use microcomputers. *Education of the Visually Handicapped, 15*(4), 135-144.

Schenk, W. A. (1985). Personal communication, December 16.

Schiffman, G., Tobin, D., & Buchanan, B. (1982). Microcomputer instruction for the learning disabled. *Journal of Learning Disabilities, 15*(9), 557-559.

Scholl, G. T. (1986). *Foundations of education for blind and visually handicapped children and youth.* New York: American Foundation for the Blind.

Scholl, G. T., & Schnur, R. (1976). *Measures of psychological, vocational, and educational functioning in the blind and visually handicapped.* New York: American Foundation for the Blind.

Schutz, R. E. (1985). Review of Stanford Achievement Test: Listening comprehension tests. In the Ninth Mental Measurements Yearbook (J. V. Mitchell, editor). Lincoln, NE: University of Nebraska Press.

Shafrath, M. R. (1986). An alternative to braille labeling. *Journal of Visual Impairment and Blindness, 80*(9), 955-956.

Shaw, D. (1974). *The development of a typing module for visually impaired pupils.* Independent study for Ed.S. Degree. Nashville: George Peabody College for Teachers.

Sheldon, W. D. (1969). Basal reader program: How do they stand today? In N. B. Smith (Ed.), *Current issues in reading* (Vol. 13). Newark, DE: International Reading.

Sloan, L., & Habel, A. (1973). Reading speeds with textbooks in large and standard print. *Sight Saving Review, 43,* 107-111

Smith, F. (1978). *Understanding reading* (2nd edition). New York: Holt, Rinehart, & Winston.

Smith, J. A. (1972). *Adventures in communication.* Boston: Allyn & Bacon.

Smits, B. W., & Mommers, M. J. (1976). Differences between blind and sighted on WISC Verbal Subtests. *New Outlook for the Blind, 70*(6), 240-246.

Sommers, V. S. (1944). *The influence of parental attitudes and social environment on the personality development of the adolescent blind.* New York: American Foundation for the Blind.

Spache, G. D. (1963). *Toward better reading.* Champaign, IL: Gaward Publications.

Spache, G. D. (1964). *Reading in the elementary school.* Boston: Allyn & Bacon.

Spache, G. D. (1972). *Diagnostic reading scales.* Monterey, CA: Test Bureau.

Spache, G. D. (1972). *The teaching of reading: Methods and results (an overview).* Bloomington: Phi Delta Kappa.

Spache, G. D. (1976a). *Diagnosing and correcting reading disabilities.* Boston: Allyn & Bacon.

Spache, G. D. (1976b). *Investigating the issues of reading disabilities.* Rockleigh, NJ: Allyn.

Spache, G. D., & Spache, E. B. (1973). *Reading in the elementary school.* Rockleigh, NJ: Allyn.

Spungin, S. J. (1977). *Competency based curriculum for teachers of the visually handicapped: A national study.* New York: American Foundation for the Blind.

Stark, M. L. (1970). Restoration and habilitation of handwriting skills to adults in a rehabilitation center setting. *New Outlook for the Blind, 64*(10), 330-339.

Steele, N. W. (1969). Learning by blind children of low ability: The relative effectiveness of reading and listening. Unpublished doctoral dissertation, George Peabody College for Teachers.

Stocker, C. S. (1963). A new approach to teaching handwriting to the blind. *New Outlook for the Blind, 57*(6), 208-210.

Stocker, C. S. (1970). *Modern methods of teaching braille.* Louisville: American Printing House for the Blind.

Stocker, C. S., & Walton, M. J. (1967). Exploring a more efficient method of teaching braille. *New Outlook for the Blind, 61*(5), 151-154.

Stone, A. A. (1964). Consciousness: Altered levels in blind retarded children. *Psychosomatic Medicine, 26*(1), 14-19.

Strauss, A., & Kephart, N. C. (1955). *Psychopathology and education of the brain-injured child (Vol. 2): Progress in theory and clinic.* New York: Grune and Stratton.

Swallow, R. M. (1981). Fifty assessment instruments commonly used with blind and partially seeing individuals. *Journal of Visual Impairment and Blindness, 75*(2), 65-72.

Sykes, K. S. (1971). A comparison of the effectiveness of standard print and large print in facilitating the reading skills of visually impaired students. *Education of the Visually Handicapped, 3*(4), 97-106.

Takemoto, Y. (1964). Script writing training at HoOpono. *New Outlook for the Blind, 58*(2), 61-62.

Telesensory Systems, Inc. (1978). Efficient Optacon reading. In *Optacon Teacher Seminar.* Palo Alto, CA: Telesensory Systems.

Tennessee School for the blind (1877). *175h Bienniel Report* to the 14th General Assembly of the State of Tennessee. Nashville: Tavel, Eastman, and Howell.

Torgesen, J. K. (1986). Computers and cognition in reading: A focus on decoding fluency. *Exceptional Children, 53*(2), 157-162.

Truan, M. B. (1978). *The effects of instructional feedback on the correct oral reading rate of visually impaired students.* Doctoral dissertation, George Peabody College for Teachers, Nashville, TN.

Tuttle, D. W. (1972). A comparison of three reading media for the blind. *Education of the Visually Handicapped, 4*(2), 40-44.

Umsted, R. G. (1970). *Improvement of braille reading through code recognition training.* Doctoral dissertation, George Peabody College for Teachers. Ann Arbor, MI, University Microfilms, No. 71-4255.

Van Cleve, E. M. (1916). How should we teach the partially sighted? *24th Bienniel Convention,* American Instructors for the Blind, Halifax, Nova Scotia.

Vander Kolk, C. J. (1981). *Assessment and planning with the visually impaired.* Baltimore, MD: University Park Press.

Vellutino, F. R., & Scanlon, D. M. (1986). Experimental evidence for the effects of instructional bias on word identification. *Exceptional Children, 53*(2). 145-155.

Warren, D. H. (1984). *Blindness and early childhood development.* New York: American Foundation for the Blind.

Weiss, J. (1980). Braille and limited language skills. *Journal of Visual Impairment and Blindness. 74*(2), 81-83.

Weiss, J., & Weiss, J. (1978). Teaching handwriting to the congentially blind. *Journal of Visual Impairment and Blindness, 72*(7), 281-283.

Wepman, J. (1973). *Auditory discrimination test.* Chicago: Language Research Association.

Wheeler, J. (1970). Teaching the concept of the diagonal during handwriting lessons for the congentially blind. *New Outlook for the Blind, 64*(8), 249-255.

Whelan, R. J. (1974). In J. M. Kauffman & C. D. Lewis (Eds.), *Teaching children with behavior disorders: Personal perspectives.* Columbus, OH: Charles E. Merrill.

White, M., & Miller, S. R. (1983). Dyslexia: A term in search of a definition. *The Journal of Special Education, 17*(1).

Wilson, L. R. (1985). Large scale learning disability identification: The reprieve of a concept. *Exceptional Children, 52*(1), 44-51.

Witt, J. C. (1985). *Review of Brigance Inventory of Basic Skills.* In Ninth Mental Measurements Yearbook (J. V. Mitchell, editor). Lincoln, NB: Univeristy of Nebraska Press.

Wood, T. D. (1981). Patterns of listening and reading skills in visually handicapped students. *Journal of Visual Impairment and Blindness, 75*(5), 215-218.

Wormsley, D. P. (1981). Hand movement training in braille reading. *Journal of Visual Impairment and Blindness, 75*(8), 327-331.

Appendices

Appendix A

220 Basic Word Sight Vocabulary

Preprimer	Primer	First	Second	Third
1. the	45. when	89. many	133. know	177. don't
2. of	46. who	90. before	134. while	178. does
3. and	47. will	91. must	135. last	179. got
4. to	48. more	92. through	136. might	180. united
5. a	49. no	93. back	137. us	181. left
6. in	50. if	94. years	138. great	182. number
7. that	51. out	95. where	139. old	183. course
8. is	52. so	96. much	140. year	184. war
9. was	53. said	97. your	141. off	185. until
10. he	54. what	98. may	142. come	186. always
11. for	55. up	99. well	143. since	187. away
12. it	56. its	100. down	144. against	188. something
13. with	57. about	101. should	145. go	189. fact
14. as	58. into	102. because	146. came	190. through
15. his	59. than	103. each	147. right	191. water
16. on	60. them	104. just	148. used	192. less
17. be	61. can	105. those	149. take	193. public
18. at	62. only	106. people	150. three	194. put
19. by	63. other	107. Mr.	151. states	195. thing
20. I	64. new	108. how	152. himself	196. almost
21. this	65. some	109. too	153. few	197. hand
22. had	66. could	110. little	154. house	198. enough
23. not	67. time	111. state	155. use	199. far
24. are	68. these	112. good	156. during	200. took
25. but	69. two	113. very	157. without	201. head
26. from	70. may	114. make	158. again	202. yet
27. or	71. then	115. would	159. place	203. government
28. have	72. do	116. still	160. American	204. system
29. an	73. first	117. own	161. around	205. better
30. they	74. any	118. see	162. however	206. set
31. which	75. my	119. men	163. home	207. told
32. one	76. now	120. work	164. small	208. nothing
33. you	77. such	121. long	165. found	209. night
34. were	78. like	122. get	166. Mrs.	210. end
35. her	79. our	123. here	167. thought	211. why
36. all	80. over	124. between	168. went	212. called
37. she	81. man	125. both	169. say	213. didn't
38. there	82. me	126. life	170. part	214. eyes
39. would	83. even	127. being	171. once	215. find
40. their	84. most	128. under	172. general	216. going
41. we	85. made	129. never	173. high	217. look
42. him	86. after	130. day	174. upon	218. asked
43. been	87. also	131. same	175. school	219. later
44. has	88. did	132. another	176. every	220. knew

Source: Dale D. Johnson, "The Dolch List Reexamined," *The Reading Teacher* 24 (February, 1971). pp. 455-456. The 220 most frequent words in the Kucera-Francis corpus.

Appendix B

Behavioral Objectives of the Braille Code

THE BEHAVIORAL Objectives of the Braille Code provide a framework from which to determine a student's mastery of braille through both reading and writing. Mastery of the code is broken into six grade levels, first through sixth grades. At each grade level words and contracted forms to be mastered are listed for reading, spelling and writing. The inclusion of the performance expectations for spelling and writing are to insure that braille skills are evaluated in each of the language arts areas.

The specific objectives at each grade level were derived from: 1) an analysis of high frequency word lists, and 2) an analysis of the vocabularies of common reading series available in braille. This information, combined with teacher experience of student progress over many years resulted in braille objectives at each elementary grade level. The Behavioral Objectives of the Braille Code are designed to aid a teacher in assessing a student's braille skills against the many skills he will need to communicate proficiently with braille. Perhaps more important, the braille code objectives will assist the teacher in setting instructional goals and organizing daily teaching lessons.

An accurate knowledge of the many components of the braille code is essential to adequate word attack skills, rate and comprehension of reading material, and effectiveness in written expression. Attainment of the following behavioral objectives at each level of development should insure the necessary proviciency for the efficient use of the code. At each level the teacher should check the objectives for all preceding levels and provide any further instruction or remediation that seems needed for any student. These levels are based on the Dolch graded list (Dolch, 1943) and should be used as a guide for determination of the reading grade level of the child. Since basal readers are largely based on this graded list or comparable lists, the teacher should find these objectives helpful in guiding the instructional program. The student is assumed to be working on grade level. If the child is not working on grade level, the teacher should make the necessary adjustments.

By the end of the *First Grade* the student will:
1. read and write the letters of the alphabet in order presented.
2. read, write, and spell orally the following words: but can do go like not so us will it the and for in be to.

3. read, write, and give the full spelling of the following part-word signs: ed ing ow ar en.
4. read the contracted forms for the following words: from have that very as with of this day father here had know mother one some work.

By the end of the *Second Grade,* the student will:

1. read, write, and spell orally: from have just more that as you this out still cannot ever name part time under upon.
2. read, write, and give the full spelling of all upper, one-cell and part-word signs: and ar ble ch ed er for ing ou ow of sh st th the wh with.
3. recognize and use correctly in written work the capital, period, and question mark.

By the end of the *Third Grade,* the student will:

1. read, write, and spell orally the following words: every people quite rather very many right work word world there where ought through these those whose their shall child which was were into by.
2. read and write the following lower, part-word signs: ea bb cc dd ff gg.
3. state orally and apply the rule that the double-letter signs and the sign for "ea" must be used only in the middle of words.
4. apply the rule that no additional letters may be added to any alphabet word sign unless those letters are separated from the sign by a hyphen or an apostrophe.
5. recognize and write exclamation mark and the apostrophe.
6. recognize and give the full spelling for the following short-form words: about after afternoon again against also almost always because before below could friend first good him himself herself little letter myself much must said such today tonight tomorrow would it itself your.
7. use the slate and stylus to write his/her own name and all the letters of the alphabet.

By the end of the *Fourth Grade,* the student will:

1. read, write, and spell: question rather lord young.
2. read, write, and give the full spelling of all final-letter signs: ound ance ence ong ful sion tion ation less ness ment ount ally ity.

3. read, write, and give the full spelling of the following part-word signs: be com con dis.
4. recognize the letter sign and explain orally the reason for its use.
5. recognize the quotation marks, hyphen, comma, and dash and write each correctly when dictated within a sentence.
6. read the following short-form words and give the full spelling of each: above across afterward already blind behind beside between children o'clock paid quick should great.
7. use the slate and stylus to write his/her name, date, and at least one dictated sentence.

By the end of the *Fifth Grade,* the student will:
1. read, write and spell: character spirit knowledge.
2. recognize and write correctly the parentheses, semicolon, and colon when dictated within a sentence.
3. use the quotation marks correctly in independent writing.
4. state orally and apply the rule which the lower signs for "to," "into," and "by" may not be used at the end of line, or immediately before any mark of puntuation.
5. apply the rule that, when it is necessary to divide a word at the end of a line, that division must be made between syllables and no contraction that would overlap those syllables may be used.
6. apply the rule that the sign for "one" may not be used when a syllable division falls between the "o" and the "n," but that otherwise the sign is used freely.
7. apply the rule that the sign for "part" may be used in any word with the exception of any form of the word "partake."
8. apply the rule that most of the initial-letter signs may not be used as part-word signs unless they retain their original sounds as words.
9. state and apply the rule that lower, whole-word signs may not be used in direct contact with any mark of punctuation.
10. state and apply the rule that, when the same amount of space is saved, a one-cell sign is used instead of a two-cell sign.
11. state orally and apply the rule that, when the same amount of space is saved, an upper sign is used instead of a lower sign.
12. read, write, and spell the following short-form words: altogether although braille beneath beyond either neither oneself ourselves together themselves yourself yourselves.

13. use the slate and stylus to write his/her name, date, and an independent paragraph of at least three sentences.

By the end of the *Sixth Grade,* the student will:

1. read, write, and give the full spelling of the following short-form words: according deceive deceiving conceive conceiving declare declaring immediate necessary perhaps perceive perceiving receive receiving rejoice rejoicing thyself.

2. explain orally that the italic sign in braille indicates that the same item in print is either underlined or appears in a special kind of type.

3. apply the rule that when three words or less are italicized one italic sign is used before each word, but when four or more words are italicized two italic signs are used before the first word and one italic sign before the last word.

4. state and apply the rule that the part-word signs for "be," "con," and "dis" may be used only for the first syllable of a word or a new line, but the sign for "com" may be used for the first three letters of a word or a new line.

5. state and apply the rule that no contraction may be used to cross the division between a prefix and a root word or the two parts of a compound word.

6. state and apply the rule that short-form words may be used as part-word contractions if they retain their original meaning, but they must not be used as parts of proper names.

7. use the slate and stylus to take a spelling test from dictation, to take brief notes, and to write an independent paragraph.

Appendix C

Word Identification Skills
by Grade Level, K-6

THE FOLLOWING guideline is based on the child who is working on grade level. If the child is not working on grade level, it will still serve as a guide to be used with reader curriculum materials. For example, if a sixth grade child is working on fourth grade level, he/she would be expected to do the word identification skills listed at the fourth grade level.

By the end of *Kindergarten,* the student will:
1. recognize own name in print and/or braille.
2. identify at least 10 upper- and lower-case letters by name.
3. identify numbers 1-10.
4. match at least 10 capital and small letters.
5. hear differences in words differing by only one phoneme (boy/ toy).
6. name the following b d j k m n p s and z single consonant sounds in a word he/she hears.
7. name the single initial consonant sound for the name of pictures and/or objects (excluding l qu v f g h r).
8. identify when words rhyme and orally name a word to rhyme with one he/she hears.
9. have completed readiness books in braille or print.

By the end of *First Grade,* the student will:
1. recognize words with either capital or lower-case letters at the beginning of the word.
2. recognize in isolation words from the Dolch List of 220 Words in the pre-primer, primer, and first grade sections with at least 80 percent accuracy.
3. identify the names of consonants and vowels.
4. use single consonants at the beginning of the word to identify words.
5. use single consonants at the end of the word to identify words.
6. identify a single consonant sound heard in the middle of a word.
7. name the long vowel or short vowel sound in one-syllable words.

298

8. decode one-syllable words using initial consonant blends formed with s l or r and diagraphs th sh st in the final position as an aid to word identification.
9. use common consonant blends lk mp pt ch st in the final position as an aid to word identification.
10. read familiar words to which the following endings have been added: ed ing s 's er.
11. recognize compound words that are composed of two familiar words, such as: someone forget something.
12. use common word family spelling patterns to identify words: all at an en ill ake it ell.
13. utilize word configuration, length, and double letters to identify words.
14. use capitalization, punctuation, and spacing when reading as clues to meaning.
15. attempt to correct reading to produce syntactically acceptable sentences as he/she reads.
16. attempt to use the following predictable vowel pattern:

    Pattern I: If a word has only one vowel in the middle, the vowel is usually short: (hop, pet).
17. score at least 90 percent accuracy on an informal reading inventory taken from the end of the first grade reader.
18. read at least 20 words per minute on end of first grade material.
19. read contracted words formed with *not, will,* and *is:* (can't, I'll, he's).
20. read common abbreviations met in basal reader (Mr., Mrs.)

By the end of *Second Grade,* the student will:

1. recognize isolated words from the Dolch List of 220 Words in the pre-primer through second grade sections with at least 80 percent accuracy.
2. recognize familiar words to which the following endings have been added: s' est es ly en ful ness.
3. recognize all contracted words formed with *are, am* (we're, I'm).
4. use most final consonant blends (ft, ld, lt, nk, nt, ng) and diagraphs (th, sh, ch, wh) in final position to identify words.
5. apply the following predictable vowel patterns to decode (student does not have to state the pattern):

    Pattern II: If a word has two vowels and one is a final "e," the first vowel is usually long and the "e" is silent (wife, hope).

Pattern III: If any of the following six vowel pairs appear in a word, the first vowel is probably long and the second is silent (ee, ea, ow, oa, ai, ay).

Pattern IV: Vowel sounds that are neither long or short are spelled with the following patterns:
/ou/ by the letters "ou," as in "out"
        by the letters "ow," as in "now"
/oi/ by the letters "oi," as in "oi"
        by the letters "oy," as in "boy"
/er/ by the letters "ur," as in "fur"
        by the letters "er," as in "her"
        by the letters, "ir," as in "sir"
/o/ by the letters "or," as in "port"

6. utilize additional common word families to identify words by rhyming (ight, ought, air, ound).

7. use the generalization for the consonant and vowel sounds of "y" (as a consonant in the initial position and as a vowel elsewhere in the word).

8. use the letters which follow "c" or "g" in a word as clues about the alternative sounds of "c" and "g" in words (c = /s/, g = /j/) when followed by "e," "i," or "y," as in circus and giant.

9. utilize consonant patterns of three letters (thr, str, spr, spl) to identify words.

10. recognize root words to which known endings are added when the root is from the current reading series.

11. match equivalent phonemes in words which show the same sound with different spellings for all phonemes taught:
(oy in boy matches oi in oil)
(j in juice matches g in gym)

12. read initials and abbreviations for common proper nouns and titles (Dr., Jan., Wed., U.S.A.).

13. read words to which the following prefixes are added: un-, re-.

14. score at least 90 percent accuracy on an informal reading inventory taken from the end of the second grade reader.

15. read at no less than 30 words per minute on late second grade material.

16. use the following syllabication guides to decode:

Guide I: Every syllable has at least one vowel letter and only one vowel sound.

Guide II: Prefixes and suffices usually form separate syllable.

By the end of *Third Grade,* the student will:

1. recognize isolated words drawn from the entire Dolch List of 220 Basic Words with at least 90 percent accuracy.
2. recognize familiar words to which the following suffixes have been added: -less, -ity, -ment, -ble.
3. recognize familiar words to which the following prefixes have been added: a-, ex-, be-, dis-, in-.
4. decode with silent letter patterns: kn-, wr-, gn-.
5. read all word contractions presented in basal series.
6. read all compound words presented in basal series.
7. identify known root word when affixes have been added which changed the spelling of the root by: dropping the final "e," doubling the final consonant, or "c," changing the "y" to "i" before adding a suffix beginning with a vowel.
8. use vowel Patterns I-III, as well as the following to decode words:

   Patterns IV: Vowel sounds that are neither long nor short are spelled with the following patterns:
   /u/ by the letter "u," as in "put"
      by the letters "oo," as in "book"
   /u/ by the letters "oo," as in "boot"
      by the letters "ew," as in "new"
   /o/ by the letters "al," as in "fall"
      by the letters "aw," as in "straw"
   /a/ by the letters "ai," as in "fair"
      by the letters "are," as in "care"
   /r/ by the letters "ar," as in "car"

9. use the following syllabication guides in addition to those previously learned to identify words:

   Guide III: Consonant blends and diagraphs are not divided (ch, str, bl).

   Guide IV: When there are two consonants between two vowels (V/CV), try dividing between the consonants and giving the first vowel a short sound (chimney).

   Guide V: When there is one consonant between two vowels (V/CV), try dividing after the first vowel and giving that vowel a long sound (pa-per).

10. correctly mark primary accented syllable using the generalization that the first syllable is accented in words without prefixes (ta'ble), and the second syllable is accented in words with prefixes (unha'py).

11. decode independently all regularly spelled words using sound-symbol relationships for initial and final consonants, consonant clusters and diagraphs, and for patterns of short, long, controlled, and variant vowels as measured by scoring at least 90 percent accuracy on tests over Part I and Part II of Hegge, Kirk, and Kirk.

12. match equivalent phonemes in words which show the same sound with different spellings for all vocabulary words presented

    ("kn" in know - the "n" in snap)

    ("ough" in thought - the "oe" in toe)

13. score at least 90 percent accuracy on an informal reading inventory taken from the end of the third grade reader.

14. read at no less than 45 words per minute on late third grade material.

By the end of the *Fourth Grade,* the student will:

1. use syllabication Guides I-V and add:

    Guide VI: If a word ends in "-le," the consonant before the "le" is part of the last syllable (ta-ble, bat-tle).

    Guide VII: Endings that form syllables are usually unaccented (run'ning).

2. use additional suffixes to decode successfully:

    (-ward, -ous, -ious, -eous, -ible, -ic, -ish, -ant, -ent, -ane, -ance, -ence, -wise, -ling, -ure, -tion, -sion, -action).

3. use additional prefixes to decode successfully (mis-, anit-, non-, com-, con-, super-, tri-, sub-, post-, ab-, trans-, em-, de-, inter-, ex-, ob-, per-).

4. syllabicate words and mark correctly the primary and secondary stress.

5. decode independently using consonant and vowel patterns as measured by a score of 95 percent on test over Part I-II of Hegge, Kirk, and Kirk, 19).

6. decode using phonemic patterns and prefixes and suffixes as demonstrated by scoring 90 percent accuracy on the test of Part III of Hegge, Kirk, and Kirk, 19).

7. use decoding skills to read in content areas of social studies, English, math, and science.
8. score at least 90 percent accuracy on an informal reading inventory taken from the end of the fourth grade reader.
9. read at no less than 50 words per minute on late fourth grade material.

By the end of the *Fifth Grade,* the student will:

1. use all previously acquired decoding skills to identify vocabulary in content areas of social studies, English, math, and science.
2. expand known prefixes and suffixes to match the vocabulary of content area materials.
3. score at least 90 percent accuracy on an informal reading inventory taken from the end of the fifth grade reader.
4. read at least 60 words per minute on late fifth grade material.

By the end of the *Sixth Grade,* the student will:

1. use phonics, structural analysis, and content clues to independently identify new vocabulary in content areas.
2. expand known prefixes and suffixes to match the vocabulary of content area materials.

Prefixes

Prefix:	Meaning:
ab	from, away
an	without, not
ad	to, toward
ante	before
bi	two, twice
circum	around
de	from, down from
dis	apart, not
dia	through, around
ex	out of, from
im	not, in
il, un, in, ir	into, not
inter	between
in, en	in, into, among
intro	within, against
mis	wrong, wrongly
non	non
pan	whole, all
per	fully, through

Suffixes

Suffix:	Meaning:
able, ible	capable of being
acy,ace,	
ancy, ance	state of being
an, ean, ian	one, who
age	relating to act
	or condition
ant	n. -one who-
	adj, being
er, ar	relating to, like
ary	n. -one who-
	(place where)
	adj. -relating to
ante	one who is little
en	made
ence	state of quality
ent	adj. -being
	n. -one who
full	full of
fy, ify	to make

Prefix:	Meaning:	Suffix:	Meaning:
peri	around, about	hood	state, condition
post	after, behind	ic	made of, like
pre	before	ice	that which
pro	for, in front of		quality or state
re	back, again	id	being in a condition of
semi	half, partly	ion	act or state of being
sub	under	ize, ise	to make
super	over, above	ist, ite	one who
trans	beyond, across	ity, ty	state relating to
tri	three, thrice	ive	
un	not		
		ment	act or state of being
		ness	state of being
		or, ar, er	one who, that
		ory	which
		ose, ous	abounding in
		some	full of
		ward	turning to, indirection
		y	like or full of

3. fully utilize all consonant sound symbol patterns to decode, including all single consonants, consonant clusters, and consonant diagraphs in initial, medial, and final positions in a word.
4. show mastery of predictable vowel patterns to decode.
5. demonstrate full mastery of guides for syllabication and ability to try different syllabication possibilities to identify words.
6. demonstrate mastery of guides for placing accents and ability to shift the accent systematically to identify the word.
7. score at least 90 percent accuracy on an informal reading inventory drawn from a sixth grade science and/or social studies text at a rate of at least 70 words per minute.

Word identification skills essential for promotion to each grade level were drawn from the following sources:

1. *Barbe Reading Skills Check List* - Levels K-6
2. *Remedial Reading Drills* - Hegge, Kirk, and Kirk
3. *The New Basic Readers Series* - Scott, Foresman and Company
4. *Ginn 360 Reading Series*
5. *Patterns Reading Series* -American Printing House
6. *Dolch List of 220 Basic Words*
7. *80 Objectives for the Tennessee Proficiency Test*

8. *Student Expectations in the Basic Skills* - K-6 - State of Tennessee, 1978
9. Scope and Sequence Skills List-Word Attck from *Teaching Students with Learning Problems* - Mercer & Mercer, 1981

Compiled by Language Arts Committee, 1982-83
Tennessee School for the Blind

Appendix D

Mechanics of Braille Reading

MAXFIELD (1928) was one of the first to emphasize good mechanics in braille reading. Children may be penalized by the using of fingers and hands in a manner which slows or retards the reading process. Excessive up and down movements, undue pressure on the fingertips, poor posture, incorrect position of the book, and many other factors can cause reading problems among blind children. The mechanics checklist in the Appendix can be used by the teacher to diagnose any special problems of the child. The checklist deals with problems with the fingers, hands, wrists, body position, lines, vision, book position, and room atmosphere. Suggestions for dealing with these problems are listed below.

Mechanics Checklist

1. The pupil reads with
   a. fingers only
   b. fingers and remaining vision
   c. fingers for braille, but uses vision for pictures and objects
2. The pupil reads with
   a. right hand
   b. left hand
   c. either hand
   d. both hands
3. The pupil uses both hands in such a manner that
   a. the left hand finds the next line
   b. the right hand finds the next line
   c. both hands move together in a parallel motion
   d. the right hand starts the next line before finishing the preceding line with the left hand
   e. the left hand starts the next line before finishing the preceding line with the right hand
4. The student holds his fingers so that
   a. the fingers are perpendicular to the page
   b. the fingers are almost parallel to the page
   c. the fingers make an acute angle with the page

5. The student reads with
   a. index finger only
   b. both index fingers
   c. index and second fingers
   d. index and second fingers of both hands
   e. other combinations (specify) _____
6. The pupil holds his book
   a. approximately parallel to the desk
   b. slanted to the right
   c. slanted to the left
   d. on his lap in front of the disk
7. The pupil moves fingers across the dots[1]
   a. stopping and rereading words or word segments frequently
   b. making frequent return sweeps
   c. at a steady rate
8. The pupil reads letters with up and down motions[2]
   a. frequently
   b. occasionally
   c. seldom if ever
9. The pupils posture when reading is
   a. excessively inclined
   b. inclined
   c. almost erect
   d. erect
10. The pupil's attitude when reading is
    a. very tense
    b. tense
    c. almost relaxed
    d. relaxed
11. The pupil's pressure on his fingertips is*
    a. variable from light to heavy
    b. heavy but uneven
    c. heavy and even
    d. less at the beginning than at the end of the line
    e. more at the end of a given paragraph
    f. light and even

---

[1]Reading of sufficient difficulty will cause problems even among experienced readers.
[2]Reading materials of sufficient difficulty will cause problems even among experienced readers.

12. The pupil reads the book
    a. above elbow level
    b. at elbow level
    c. below elbow level
13. The pupil's chair is
    a. too high
    b. too low
    c. just right for feet to rest comfortably on the floor
14. The pupil loses his place
    a. seldom if ever
    b. sometimes
    c. frequently
15. The pupil reads by
    a. attending to each letter or contraction individually
    b. grouping letters into words
    c. grouping words into phrases or sentences
16. The pupil reads orally by
    a. reading all letters before calling the word
    b. reading all but ending letters to identify words
    c. using first letters to identify words
17. The pupil's perception of dots is characterized by
    a. missed dot errors
    b. added dot errors
    c. ending dot errors
    d. no perceptual errors
18. The pupil's orientation to the braille cell is characterized by
    a. reversal errors
    b. vertical alignment problems
    c. horizontal alignment problems
    d. no orientation problems
19. The pupil's recognition of words is characterized by
    a. association errors
    b. substitution errors
    c. omission errors
    d. no recognition problems
20. The pupil's behavior during reading is characterized by
    a. head movements
    b. body rocking
    c. eye poking
    d. other mannerisms
    e. no mannerisms or unnecessary movements

21. The position of the wrists is
    a. sagging below line
    b. humped above line
    c. fairly straight in line with hands and arms
22. The pupil's silent reading is characterized by
    a. excessive oral lip movements
    b. excessive silent lip movements
    c. occasional lip movements
    d. no lip movements
23. The pupil's speed in silent reading of easy material is
    a. less than 20 words per minute
    b. 20 to 40 words per minute
    c. 40 to 60 words per minute
    d. 60 to 80 words per minute
    e. more than 80 words per minute
24. The pupil uses his remaining vision
    a. not at all
    b. for three-dimensional objects
    c. for braille reading assistance
    d. for pictures

Suggestions for the Use of the Mechanics Checklit

1. Braille readers often use vision for interpreting pictures even when they are unable to read print. The alert teacher will take advantage of any remaining vision to teach concepts with pictures and real objects. If the child is able to use remaining vision to read braille, the child will be penalized in two ways: (1) he will lose valuable time which could be devoted to print reading, and (2) he cannot become very proficient in braille reading with his fingers.

2. Research has shown that a majority of mature braille readers use both hands and that reading with both hands produces the most rapid rate of reading.

3. The return sweep in braille reading takes a considerable amount of time compared to print reading (6 or 7% of total reading time in braille reading). Good readers are characterized as those whose hands function independently of each other. Readers who read ahead with the left hand while the right hand finishes the preceding line tend to be more efficient readers.

4. The fingers should be curved comfortably, making an acute angle with the page and allowing the pads of the fingers to span the entire three-dot depth of the cell.

5. As many fingers as possible should be utilized in the reading process.
6. The book should be placed in a comfortable position. Books are usually held parallel with the edge of the table or at a slight acute angle by most good readers.
7. Smooth and steady left-right hand movements are characteristic of the good braille reader.
8. Rubbing or frequent up and down motions are characteristic of a poor reader.
9. Although posture does not seem to affect reading efficiency, a good posture is healthy for the body and unwarranted fatigue is prevented.
10. The best reading occurs in a relaxed position. The teacher can assist in developing a relaxed classroom atmosphere.
11. A light, even pressure is best for good perception of the braille dots.
12. The book should be no higher than elbow level.
13. The pupil's feet should rest comfortably on the floor.
14. The good reader seldom if ever loses his place. Are both hands being used together? The left hand can be used to hold the place at the beginning of the line if necessary.
15. Individual letter reading is characteristic of the beginning reader.
16. Reading rate can be increased by using letter and word cues to identify words before identifying each letter of the word. However, excessive errors may indicate a need to identify the complete configuration before calling the word.
17. Missed dot errors are most prevalent in words with multiple cell contractions and often indicate premature closure or arriving at a conclusion without all of the information. Ending problems are most commonly found with abbreviated words. Suggestions for teaching include: (1) use easy and meaningful materials, (2) develop anticipation span using short idea units, and (3) do not try to speed up reading rate until accuracy in perception is attained.
18. Reversals are most common in contracted word forms, and appear most often in beginning readers in the primary grades. Retracings for unfamiliar words may lead to an increase in the number of reversals. Suggestions for teaching include use of (1) good mechanics and (2) easy to read materials. Vertical alignment errors occur most frequently with lower cell contractions. A reduction in the number of lower cell contractions in the reading might help reduce errors. Horizontal alignment errors occur most often with multiple cell

contractions. A reduction in the number of multiple cell contractions can help to reduce errors.

19. Association errors occur most commonly in whole word signs. Common association errors are "did" for "do" or "quick" for "quite."

20. Mannerisms such as head movements, body rocking, and eye poking may or may not interfere with braille reading efficiency. The reduction and elimination of mannerisms can often be obtained through the provisions of more socially accepted physical activities for the child. Behavior modification procedures have been successfully used to eliminate such mannerisms often called "blindisms."

21. The child generally reads most efficiently when the wrists are fairly straight in line with hands and arms. If humping or sagging of the wrists occur, the teacher can correct the student by simply touching or lifting the wrists.

22. Speed in silent reading is difficult to obtain when the pupil is using lip movements. If lip reading occurs during silent reading, the teacher can correct the student simply by touching his upper or lower lip. Chewing gum or placing a sterile object in the mouth is sometimes used to stop lip movements.

23. Training in character and word recognition through regularly scheduled drills have proven to be an effective method of increasing speed. Other proven methods include the improvement of mechanics of reading such as using both hands independently, practice in reading short passages, and building confidence through practice in reading easy passages.

24. The use of residual vision to see pictures in books or three-dimensional objects representing concepts in the books can be very helpful to meaningful reading. The use of vision in reading braille could be an indicator that the child should read print materials.

Appendix E

Writing Tips for Reporting an Educational Assessment

General Tips for Writing: In case you forgot

1. Do not use one-sentence paragraphs.
2. Do not begin a paragraph with a pronoun.
3. Maintain the same writing tense within a sentence and within a paragraph if possible.
4. Carefully check subject/verb agreement.
5. Number pages in upper right corner with the number only.
6. A page should not begin with a single line of type.
7. A page should not end with a hyphen.
8. Use full words instead of contracted forms (did not instead of didn't).
9. If using an abbreviation, the full name of the test or work should be given first along with the abbreviation (Informal Reading Inventory — IRI).

Writing an Assessment

A. Organization

1. The most pertinent information should appear prominently on the first page (student's name, date of birth, parents names, address and phone, current educational placement, date(s) of evaluation are most important). Additional information may include a list of test materials used, previous dates of testing and results, officially identified handicaps, reading mode, and referring person or agency.
2. Organize the assessment into sections. Make use of headings to facilitate interpretation of and referal to the report. The following topics should be discussed, either as separate sections or as part of other sections.
   a. *Referral.* Briefly state who referred the child and why. Identifying the questions to be answered will guide the selection of the test to provide the requested information. Identifying the referring agency or individual will influence, to some degree, the complexity and detail in the written results.

b. *History.* Include medical information in child's records with dates of tests or diagnoses. Report only information pertinent to the educational assessment. The history should indicate major handicapping conditions with official medical diagnoses when available. The stability of the child's health should be noted. The composition of the family and educational environment and educational history are important.

c. *Overview of Results.* Include most obvious physical characteristics (age, race, social poise, reaction to testing, and work attitude). Include a statement of major findings in view of referral.

d. *Results.* The way the results section is structured will be determined by the purpose of the assessment and the tests used. If the child is functioning at a preacademic level, the major sections of the results might be motor *cognition, language,* and *socialization.* If the referee is school age, information about academic performance will be the primary focus. Reporting may be by academic areas such as *reading, listening, math,* or may include sections about *general knowledge, self help skills,* and *motor development.* A separate section about *visual functioning* may be required or use of vision may be incorporated in all topics.

e. *Discussion or Interpretation.* Interpretation may be interwoven with the results in a combined section. The purpose of each is quite different. Results are observable and measurable behaviors of the child. Interpretations are your conclusions by observing the point at which the child was unsuccessful and the manner in which he/she failed. From the results you may interpret underlying problems or delays. Once underlying problems are clearly identified, future problems can be anticipated and some teaching strategy selected to remediate or circumvent the delay.

For example many of the reading errors that Leanne made when reading individual words or words in passages involved misperceptions of the shape of the braille characters (*shaking* for *making; sule* for *single*) or involved lower signs (*to train* for *by train*). Such errors would indicate a problem with spatial concepts. An interpretation should be supported by more than one example. The pervasiveness of the problem should be identified if it is also evident in other areas—academic or developmental areas. The child's failure on a particular task may have a wide range of causes. For most skills assessed there are several examples of items testing the same concept in various ways. By comparing performance on similar items it is possible to draw specific conclusions about why the child failed. For example, if the child fails a sorting task of three colors, he may have failed because he did not understand the concept, did not understand the instructions, was distracted by too many variables, or could not differentiate color. If he could sort three different shapes or sounds, than he had the concept of sorting and his inability was in discriminating colors.

f. *Conclusions and/or Recommendations*. State the range of skills sampled such as: Leanne's highest skills were in using phonics to decode words and matching what she read to predictable sentence patterns. Her weakest skills were involved in spatial concepts as they relate to laterality, orientation, and sequencing of letters, numbers, and events. If academic scores are obtained, report the highest and lowest ranges (mid-third grade).

List recommendations and conclusions in order of importance or priority for instruction. Be specific about where to begin instruction and, if possible, the strategy or methods that might be most effective. These recommendations may become the objective for the individual education program. The labeling of an underlying problem is not of much value to many teachers. The need is for identifying materials, methods, and guides to teach the child to remediate the delay or detour the deficit. The recommendation and/or conclusions section may also contain a specific recommendation about the type of program required to provide for the recommended instruction.

g. *Signature*. Sign and date the report and identify your official position at the time of testing.

B. Writing Style

1. Describe the activities you observed in the child in behavioral terms that could be remeasured.
2. Word your statements carefully. If sentences can be taken to mean several things or there could be a different interpretation, revise the sentence.
3. Use the past tense throughout except in the "recommendations."
4. Carefully phrase the wording about what the child could do so that it has the most positive tone possible. The whole point is to identify the next skills levels to be taught which are the activities the child did not fully complete. Instead of writing "Jim could not

read fractions." You might write, "Jim read all fractions as two digit numbers."

5. Do no list scores without some interpretation of his/her performance on the test. The numerical score is not what is significant. Because a percentage or grade equivalent score is small and simple, it stands out and may receive undue attention. The tendency is to consider numerical scores as absolute. Actually, such scores fluctuate due to environmental factors such as test setting, familiarity of child with examiner, the child's physical condition, etc. The fluctuation of scores is especially common with handicapped children who were excluded from the norming population.

6. Describe the child's unsuccessful attempts which clearly illustrate why the child failed. For example, the child in the videotape of the McCarthy failed to build the house because of a lack of eye-hand coordination (motorically) rather than not understanding the task (cognitively).

7. List the tests or procedure used. If only parts are used, identify the subtest or mention that items were "selected at random" or "sampled." A list of tests may be omitted if skills are only screened for confirmation of a placement or need to retest.

Appendix F

Objectives for Written Language, K-12

THE FOLLOWING objectives for written language are skills that should be acquired by students who are achieving at grade level. It is recognized that most visually impaired children will not be functioning at grade level. However, the objectives in written language should be matched from this guide with the grade level of readers and curriculum materials which the student is able to read. These objectives for written language list skills in the areas of composition, format, capitalization, punctuation, parts of speech, subject verb agreement, synonyms, antonyms, homonyms, plurals, possessives, spelling, study skills, and creative writing. Unique objectives concerning braille are addressed in Appendix B, Behavioral Objectives for the Braille Code. Methods of assessing and teaching handwriting are described in Chapter 8.

The objectives are provided here to assist the teacher of visually impaired students in identifying the specific content of written language that is typically presented at each grade level. The teacher of visually impaired students will have a condensed view of the scope and sequence of each area of writing. The teacher may find similar and more specific information in the supplemental teaching materials that are designed to accompany the student's textbook. However, such materials may not be readily available to the vision specialist. The list of objectives may be especially helpful to the vision specialist in assessment and in selecting and sequencing objectives in preparation for the student's Individual Education Program. Within any classroom at any one grade level there may be students with skills ranging as much as two grade levels above and two grade levels below the skills listed in these objectives. The list can be especially helpful for planning instruction for these students.

By the end of *Kindergarten,* the student will:
1. recognize own name in print and/or braille.
2. print or braille own first name with appropriate capitals and lower-case letters.
3. write at least 10 lower-case letters of the alphabet.

By the end of *First Grade,* the student will:
1. print or braille full name, correctly forming all capital and lower-case letters.

2. spell pre-primer and primer words from the Dolch 220 List with a minimum of 80 percent accuracy.
3. compose a simple sentence using a capital and a period or question mark as appropriate.
4. copy the days of the week and names of numbers from one to ten.
5. write the literary numbers from one to ten.
6. when writing capitalize the word I, the first word in a sentence, and familiar proper nouns.
7. accurately copy (capitals, punctuation, spacing, and spelling) sentences of at least five words.
8. appropriately space between consecutive lines when writing.
9. begin writing on left margin.

By the end of *Second Grade,* the student will:

1. write simple sentences of at least five words from dictation, using capitals and periods and/or questions marks.
2. write the days of the week and copy the months of the year with correct spelling and capitalization.
3. use commas between the day of the month and the year.
4. capitalize:
   names of persons
   names of pets
   the days of the week and month
5. pair, and use in writing, words on grade level that are synonyms, antonyms, and homonyms.
6. correctly write, spell and capitalize significant proper nouns (classmates, teacher, parents, pets, siblings).
7. write telephone number.
8. spell pre-primer, primer and first grade words from Dolch 220 List with 80 percent accuracy.
9. use a period after numbers for items.
10. form plural nouns by adding -s.

By the end of *Third Grade,* the student will:

1. write full name, telephone number, birthday.
2. compose simple sentences using correct punctuation, capitalization, and spelling.
3. correctly compose a simple original paragraph except for title.
4. capitalize:
   greeting and closing of a note or letter

street, town, and state
titles: Mr., Mrs., Miss
places, as Fort Knox
major holidays
initials
name of school

5. use comma:
   between city and state
   after greeting and closing of friendly letter
6. use period:
   after abbreviations
   after initials
7. use all forms of end punctuation in short sentences.
8. recognize nouns, active verbs, and adjectives.
9. correctly use homonyms that are contained in speller.
10. form plural nouns by adding -s or -es.
11. write possessives of singular nouns.
12. spell basic Dolch sight words, pre-primer-second grade and common proper nouns with 80 percent accuracy.
13. write sentences from dictation, using pre-primer-through second grade Dolch words.
14. spell words from third grade speller, both in isolation and in sentences.
15. write abbreviations of commonly-used words (days of week, months of year, some titles of respect, pupil's state).
16. write signature (print students).
17. write all the months and their abbreviations.
18. follow written directions of two steps.

By the end of *Fourth Grade*, the student will:

1. recognize parts of a friendly letter:
   heading
   greeting
   body
   closing
2. compose a thank-you note.
3. handle brailler or pencil adequately to maintain straight margins for two columns on a paper.
4. write own address in correct format.

5. capitalize:

   titles: Dr., Ms.

   specific places, such as White House.
6. use comma after words in a series.
7. identify nouns, action verbs, adjectives, and adverbs in sentences.
8. correctly use homonyms contained in speller.
9. form plurals of spelling words by adding -s, -es, y to i and add -es, -f to -v and add -es or -s, or changing the form of the word.
10. write the possessive form of plural nouns ending in -s.
11. spell basic Dolch sight words on entire list.
12. spell word from fourth grade speller, both in isolation and in sentences.
13. follow written directions of at least three steps.
14. compose a simple paragraph with a title on a given topic.
15. select the correct form of comparative adjectives that are formed by adding -es or -est.

By the end of *Fifth Grade,* the student will:

1. compose an invitation and an announcement.
2. use correct form when writing a friendly letter and in writing the address on the envelope.
3. underline the titles of books.
4. capitalize titles of magazines, stories, and poems.
5. capitalize:

   names of companies, stores, and clubs

   the first word in a quotation

   names of continents, countries, and nationalities
6. use commas:

   between a direct quotation and the rest of the sentence (not split quote).

   between the day of the week and the month (Sunday, April 20) and after a date within a sentence (. . . . April 20, 1986,).

   after the city and state within a sentence (. . . Nashville, Tennessee,).
7. use quotation marks to set off a direct quotation.
8. recognize three kinds of sentences (declarative, interrogative, and exclamatory).

9. identify simple subjects and predicates; identify complete subject and predicate.
10. identify prepositions, pronouns, nouns, adjectives, and adverbs.
11. correctly use homonyms contained in speller.
12. use the correct possessive form of a singular and plural nouns in writing.
13. spell words from fifth grade speller, both in isolation and in sentences.
14. follow written 4-step directions (see p. 7).
15. write at least two paragraphs related to a topic with paragraph indentations and a centered title.

By the end of *Sixth Grade,* the student will:
1. make written summaries of any material read.
2. capitalize:
   each main topic and subtopic in an outline.
   names of events and documents, such as *Battle of New Orleans, Declaration of Independence.*
   names of school subjects which are names of nationalities.
   names of departments of govenrment, political parties, as Congress, Republican.
   all proper nouns.
3. use a period after a capital letter or Roman numeral in an outline.
4. use a comma:
   after introductory words such as *yes, no.*
   to separate the name of the person spoken to from rest of sentence.
5. use a colon:
   after greeting of a business letter.
   to write time in figures.
6. use a hyphen between syllables at the end of a line.
7. recognize present, past, and future tenses.
8. know, and use in writing, at least 50 percent of antonyms, synonyms, and homonyms contained in speller.
9. identify verbs of being, including helping verbs, as well as active verbs, nouns, adjectives, pronouns, prepositions, conjunctions, and interjections.
10. use most prefixes and suffixes found in reading when writing.

11. identify all four sentence types.
12. distinguish between complete and incomplete sentences.
13. spell words in sixth grade speller, both in isolation and in sentences.
14. recognize and delete irrelevant sentences from paragraph.
15. construct at least three paragraphs in a theme with appropriate title, indentation, margins, punctuation, and spelling.
16. use recall, sequence, and order in expressing written ideas.

By the end of *Seventh Grade,* the student will:

1. write a topic sentence.
2. write at least three paragraphs about a selected subject.
3. correctly use the comparison of adjectives in writing.
4. use subject and predicate in agreement.
5. avoid use of double negatives in writing.
6. correctly use verbs, including troublesome and irregular ones, in writing.
7. write geographical directions with appropriate capitalization.
8. keep the same tense within a paper.
9. identify all parts of speech including nouns, verbs, adverbs, adjectives, prepositions, conjunctions, interjections, and pronouns.
10. use quotations correctly in split quotations.
11. begin new paragraphs with change of speaker.
12. use comma:
    to set off exact words of speaker from rest of sentence
    to set off noun in direct address
13. recognize and *avoid* using run-on sentences.
14. correctly form singular and plural possessives.
15. spell words in seventh grade speller, both in sentences and in isolation.

By the end of the *Eighth Grade,* the student will:

1. write reasons, examples or facts to support a topic sentence.
2. choose and limit a topic.
3. fill out forms and applications.
4. write clear directions of several steps.
5. write sentences with varied structure (simple, compound, complex, and compound-complex).
6. identify gerunds and participles in addition to eight parts of speech.

7. identify direct objects, indirect objects, and adverbial phrases and clauses.
8. use quotations to set off titles of poems, songs, chapter titles, articles, and short stories.
9. italicize names of books, newspapers, and magazines.
10. use a hyphen in spelling the names of numbers from 1-29.

By the end of *Ninth Grade,* the student will:

1. write a well-organized paper of several paragraphs (topic sentences, sequence, conclusion, etc.).
2. write with at least seven different sentence patterns.
3. identify prepositional phrases used as either adjectives or adverbs.
4. use comma:
   after introductory dependent clause
   before conjunction that joins two parts of compound sentence
   to set off appositives
5. italicize name of ships, planes, and trains.

By the end of *Tenth Grade,* the student will:

1. use various methods of paragraph development:
   chronological
   definition
   spatial
   comparison and contast
   order of importance
   cause and effect
2. state a hypothesis.
3. distinguish between main and subordinate ideas.
4. use the following correct punctuation:
   dash
   hyphen
   colon preceeding an enumeration of a list of items
5. use comma to set off inserted words.

By the end of *Eleventh Grade,* the student will:

1. write essays.
2. research, organize, and write a paper compiled from books and periodicals.
3. use parallelism in phrases, clauses, sentences, and outlines.
4. use single quotation marks correctly.
5. use parentheses correctly.

By the end of *Twelfth Grade,* the student will:

1. research, organize, and write a research paper using the following: books, periodicals, interviews, and pamphlets and include title page, bibliography, and reference citations.
2. compile a personal data sheet.
3. identify figures of speech:
   metaphors
   personification
   hyperbole.
4. identify sound devices:
   alliteration
   onomatopoeia.
5. use semicolons, brackets, and ellipsis correctly.

Appendix G

Resources

Companies

A NUMBER of companies have developed as a result of the need for electronic aids for visually impaired people. Generally, these companies have as a goal to develop, manufacture, and distribute electronic aids that will eliminate some of the limitations imposed by visual impairment and blindness. Following is a list of some of the major companies that produce electronic aids and software specially designed for the visually impaired.

Raised Dot Computing
408 South Baldwin Street
Madison, Wisconsin 53703
(608) 257-9595

Street Electronics
Special Needs Division
124 West Washington
Lower Arcade
Fort Wayne, Indiana 46802
(219) 422-2424

Telesensory Systems, Inc.
P.O. Box 7455
Mountain View, CA 94039-7455
in CA: (415) 960-0920
toll-free outside CA (800) 227-8418

Triformation Systems
3102 S.E. Jay Street
Stuart, FL 33497
(305) 283-4817

VTEK (formerly VisualTek)
1625 Olympic Blvd.
Santa Monica, CA 90404
(213) 829-6841
Toll free (800) 345-2256
or from CA (800) 521-5605

Wormald Sensory Aids Cooperation
Suite 110, White Pine Office Centre
205 West Grand Avenue
Bensenville, IL 60106
(312) 766-3935

(People in mid-western states of ND, SD, NE, MN, IA, WI, IL, MI, IN, OH contact Wormald at above address. All other states contact Telesensory in CA.)

Agencies and Organizations

Agencies and organizations can be a valuable resource for gaining information about electronic aids and software to meet the needs of visually impaired students. Teachers of visually impaired students should become aware of national, state, and local agencies that can provide information and assistance.

American Foundation for the Blind
15 West 16th Street
New York, NY 10011

American Printing House for the Blind
1839 Frankfort Avenue
P.O. Box 6085
Louisville, KY 40206

National Federation for the Blind
Committee on Evaluation of Technology
1800 Johnston Street
Baltimore, MD 21230
(301) 659-9314

SPEECH Enterprises
Special Computer Resources
P.O. Box 7986
Houston, TX 77270-7986

Universities

A number of colleges and universities have received grants during the past few years to develop, adapt, and/or field test electronic aids and access equipment for microcomputers for the visually impaired. Some have manuals for teacher and student use as a result of their efforts. A number of programs offer college level training for teachers of the visually impaired in the area of technology.

**Trace Research and Development Center
on Communication, Control & Computer Access
for Handicapped Individuals**
University of Wisconsin-Madison
1500 Highland Avenue
Madison, Wisconsin 53705-2280
(608) 262-5408

Rehabilitation Centers for the Blind

Rehabilitation centers for the visually impaired are a valuable resource for gaining information and skills relevant to the use of electronics aid with visually impaired students. Students may be able to attend specific courses designed to teach them the use of electronic aids.

The Carrol Center for the Blind
770 Center Street
Newton, MA 02158
(617) 969-6200

Residential Schools for the Blind

Generally, residential schools for the blind have more electronic aids than local educational agencies due to their greater populations of blind students. Personnel at residential schools may be a valuable source of information regarding the use of various devices.

Individuals

There are numerous professionals in the field of visual impairment that have gained expertise with electronic aids for the visually impaired, and especially with microcomputers and the access technology. Many of these people are available to make presentations at workshops and inservice training activities. Some are willing to answer questions and concerns by telephone. Lists of experts are available from a variety of resources (e.g., SPEECH Enterprises of Houston, Texas, and Trace Center of University of Wisconsin-Madison). Names of experts can also be obtained by calling the various national and state agencies that deal specifically with the needs of the visually impaired, state departments of education, universities, residential schools, and local educational agencies.

Magazines and Newsletters

Closing the Gap Newsletter
Bud Hagen, Editor
P.O. Box 68
Henderson, MN 56044

Journal of Visual Impairment and Blindness
American Foundation for the Blind
15 West 16th Street
New York, NY 10011

(Has a specific section called Random Access that deals with microcomputers in each issue.)

Raised Dot Computing (Newsletter)
408 South Baldwin Street
Madison, WI 53703
General: (608) 257-9595
Techincal: (608) 257-8833

AUTHOR INDEX

SUBJECT INDEX